F B C

The Full Bladder Club

One man's encounter with radiation therapy
for prostate cancer

Helmut Stefan

Science & Humanities Press
Saint Charles Missouri USA

ISBN 978-1-59630-095-8

LCCN 2015937008

I hope that you will find the following pages to be informative and entertaining. And if one passage or another elicits a little chuckle from you, well, that would really make me happy.

The names of all persons have been changed to protect their privacy.

Graphics Credits

Linear Accelerator © Stockage | Dreamstime.com

File ID: 45053737

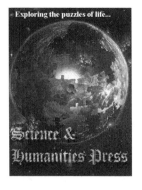

𝕾cience & 𝕳umanities 𝕻ress

Saint Charles Missouri USA

Health is the greatest gift,
Contentment is the greatest wealth,
Faithfulness is the best relationship.

Buddha

Dear Barbara,

I am glad that you are
one of the lively, witty and
charming women in my life.

Sincerely,

H. Stefan

This book is dedicated to everyone who, directly or indirectly, has been affected by the ravages of cancer, and to the men and women who have dedicated their lives to combat this insidious disease.

The Phone Call

I am now an alumnus of the FBC. My membership began about nine weeks ago, and I look back to those nine weeks with very mixed feelings. Mind you, I did not want to be a member of the FBC group. I could never imagine that I would ever be part of that bunch. But here I am – and this is how I spent the last nine weeks of my life.

It all began about four months ago with that phone call from Dr. Bauer. It was exactly 9:01 pm. I know this because the nine o'clock news had just begun. When I saw the name on the caller ID, I turned the TV to mute and said, "Hi, Dr. Bauer." The fact that he called at this hour did not surprise me. He had done this many times before, usually after he had received the results of my blood tests, and usually the news was good, or, at least, not bad. Cholesterol slightly elevated, blood sugar could be a little lower, this or that borderline; watch your weight a little more. See you at our next appointment. That is what I expected to hear this time, too.

And he began just as I had expected, "I have just received your blood work results and everything looks pretty good." Good, I thought, the usual admonitions, thank you for calling, see you next time.

But he continued, "I do, however, have some concerns about the PSA level." This statement made me sit up and listen. For all these years now, there had been no problem. Always at 2.5, and the office prostate exam showed no abnormalities. So this couldn't be too bad, I thought.

"The PSA number has gone up to four," he continued. "Normally, physicians become alarmed if the number doubles, which yours has not, yet I feel we should take a closer look."

"Okay," I replied, "what do you propose?"

"I think we should do another test, the protein free test (I think that's what he said). That will zero in more specifically on the PSA situation. I will give you a referral to have this test done. It's just better to play it safe."

I had the blood test done a few days later and shortly thereafter I heard from Dr. Bauer again, and just about at the same time of night as before. He came right to the point.

"The blood test shows that there is a significant change in the PSA, and I think you should have a prostate biopsy done. I want you to call Dr. Delgado's office and make an appointment to see him. He is an excellent urologist and will know how to proceed with this matter. OK?"

I thanked him for calling me so soon and said good night.

I sat in Dr. Delgado's office a week later. He greeted me cordially and had a bunch of papers in his hand. We sat down and he began to go over the various numbers on the report and explained what they could possibly indicate. Then he told me that he definitely agreed with Dr. Bauer that I should have a biopsy done.

"Not now," he said, "we'll do that next week. But first, let me check your prostate." I knew the drill (pun intended). I pulled down my pants and bent over the table. "Not enlarged," he told me, "but fairly hard on the sides."

Okay, I thought, good to know. After I had put myself back together again, he shook my hand and said,

"Just stop at the front desk a minute. They will give you a time for when we can do the biopsy."

My wife and I were back a week later. Within minutes, I was asked to come into the back. Here there were numerous doors leading to various treatment, consultation and evaluation rooms. A nurse took me to one of these rooms and asked me to bare my right butt cheek, so that she could give me an injection. Although I am sure that she was careful and very professional about giving me the shot, it was one of the most painful injections I have ever had in my life. And I still felt a pain in that region weeks later. A male technician now came into the room, introduced himself, and told me to strip down from the waist. As I did, he pointed out that he really liked my sandals.

"Thanks," I replied, "these are Ecco's and I bought them just a few weeks ago in a picturesque town in the Bavarian Alps."

Then I had to get on the examining table, lie on my left side and pull my legs up in a fetal position. Dr. Delgado entered the room.

"Looks like we're ready to go." I thought to myself, you might be ready, but I'm not sure about me.

I held on tight to the metal bar on the side of the table and closed my eyes. Then, I felt it, and it was not a good feeling. Not only did it (whatever it was) go ever more deeply into me, it was also shifted from side to side to what I considered to be close to the stretching limit of that orifice.

"Here we go," said the doctor. I heard a click-click, and then a sharp pain shot through my body. Pause. Click-click. Another sharp pain shot through me. The object then

3

moved as if it was looking for something specific (which it probably was). Click-click. Pain. More movement. Stop. Click-click. More movement. Stop. Click-click. By now both of my hands were tightly clasped around the metal bar. Click-click. Ouch, that one hurt even more than the others - painful stretching movement - click-click. I stopped counting. The probing continued and so did the click-clicks. Finally, the doctor said, "One more and we're all done." I breathed a sigh of relief. The click-click came, pain, then a quick feeling of something being withdrawn. Several wipes by the technician, and it was all over. Dr. Delgado told me that the results would be sent to my doctor.

Dr. Bauer called me a few days later. The biopsy results showed that out of the twelve samples, five were cancerous, three benign, but two were active. I think he was surprised when I asked him about the Gleason number.

"I see you have investigated this. That's good." He paused a few seconds and then said, "Yes, I have it here. Your Gleason number is three plus three, so that's a six."

The reason I knew about this number is because a friend of mine has prostate cancer and his Gleason number was ten. He had his prostate and lymph nodes removed.

"As you know," Dr. Bauer continued, "the Gleason number indicates the aggressiveness of the cancer. A six is right in the middle, and in your case, the cancer has not spread anywhere. So, this is definitely treatable. I'm sure Dr. Delgado will call you for an appointment to discuss treatment options."

And so it went. I met with Dr. Delgado a few days later. He made every effort to relieve me of any anxiety I may have had. Then he explained, in laymen terms, the three basic methods of treatment - external radiation therapy (radiation applied by a linear accelerator); internal radiation therapy (implantation of radioactive seeds); total removal of the gland.

Of course, he was more specific than that and explained the various pros and cons of each treatment method. When he was finished, I asked him, "So, what's the best plan for me?"

He said, "For your particular case, I recommend the most conservative approach, and that is the external radiation method. It is painless and offers you the best opportunity to continue your life in your normal way." (I don't remember if those were his exact words, but that is pretty much the message I picked up).

"OK," I said, "so what's the next step?"

"I will contact Dr. Sinclair's office; he is a radiation oncologist, right here downstairs in this building. He will take over from here and discuss all of the details with you."

I was back in the same building within a week, but this time I went right past the receptionist and the people in the waiting room. I took the elevator one floor down and introduced myself to the receptionist. Interestingly enough, she asked me to look into a camera and took my picture. "That's for your ID," she told me. Soon thereafter I was escorted into the back and asked to wait in one of the examining rooms. Dr. Sinclair appeared shortly and reviewed my case with me. The gist of it was that he agreed with Dr. Delgado, that radiation therapy was the best treatment method for me. Then he explained to me the three steps necessary before the therapy could actually begin.

Visit 1: Implantation of three tiny gold pieces into the prostate gland; this is the fiducial marker placement procedure. This assists in the proper prostate alignment during the radiation treatment.

Visit 2: CT simulation. This allows visualization of the treatment area and makes it possible for the physicist and the physician to make a specific treatment plan for the patient. At that time, a mixture of contrast dye and water will be injected into the bladder. Finally, a mold will be taken of the legs, which will then be used at each treatment to assure the correct body alignment.

Visit 3: Tattooing. Based upon the markings that were placed on the body during the previous visit, ink is now inserted just under the skin (the size of a freckle, I was told) in exactly the same spots. These permanent "tattoos" assure the correct body position during each treatment.

"Before you leave," Dr. Sinclair stated, "let me just do one more check of your prostate." After assuming the same position as before, he continued, "Rather firm." He then he told me to stop at the desk down the hall where I would be given an appointment and instructions for the fiducial marker placement procedure. I was just ready to leave the room when he continued, "During this procedure you will probably not consider me to be your friend." I understood this warning all too well, but I smiled anyway, as I shook his hand and left the room.

A week later, my wife and I were back. Again, I was led to the same examining room and the male assistant (I don't remember his name) asked me to strip from the waist down. He had me lie on my left side on the exam table and gave me a shot in the right buttock. "This will make it a little easier," he said. Shortly thereafter Dr. Sinclair arrived and said, "Looks like we're all set. This won't take long."

It's true, it didn't take all that long, but this was an entirely different kind of pain. Again, some object went into me and poked around. The doctor said, "Here comes number one." That was followed by a pain, which clearly stemmed from a sharp object slowly being pushed into living tissue. Fortunately, that did not last very long. After a little more probing, I heard him say, "Here comes number two," and the pain was just as intense. "OK," he said, "we're almost done because here comes number three." By now, I think I was close to having tears in my eyes, but then it was indeed over. Clean up; slowly back into a sitting position, one step down, clothes back on. That wasn't fun, but if it was necessary, well, a man's gotta do what a man's gotta do.

My wife and I were back a week later for the three procedures, which were to follow next: the scan with the body markings, the injection of a contrast dye and water into the bladder, and the making of the mold for the legs. After a short wait in the waiting room, a young lady asked me to come with her. She took me to one of the examination rooms. She told me that her name was Pat and that she was the chief therapist. We sat down across from each other and then she began. "First, I will tell you what we are going to do today. Then Dr. Arnold will come in and go over the consent for radiation therapy form with you. Then I will come back and take you to the room where the procedures will be performed." I nodded. She looked at me and went on, "First, I will disinfect the tip of your penis. Then, a small, very short tube will be inserted into your penis through which a water and dye solution will be injected into your bladder. I will then place a lightweight clamp at the base of your penis to prevent the injected liquid from leaking out." I nodded. Now, female doctors have treated me before, including the infamous scrotum-holding-cough test, and a very tall and slender doctor, with correspondingly thin fingers, had done a prostate exam on me. None of that bothered me. As a matter of fact, I have always found the treatment by female doctors to be very sensitive and highly professional. However, this sudden triple penis barrage did take me slightly by surprise. I had absolutely expected that male doctors and male assistants would do all this work, the way I had experienced it before. This sudden revelation definitely added a slightly different touch to the whole situation. She then also explained the scanning procedure, the marks that were to be drawn on my skin, and the making of the molds in which my legs would be placed during each radiation session. "OK?" she smiled. "I will now ask Dr. Arnold to come in to go over the consent form with you, and then, I will take you to the room where we will do the procedures. She smiled again and I smiled back.

Dr. Arnold entered the room almost immediately, introduced himself and shook my hand. He had a form with him that he handed me. It was the consent form. "Are there any questions?" he asked.

"No," I replied. I had read all about the risks of the procedure before and saw nothing new on the form. I was willing to sign.

The doctor looked at the form, which had my name on the top line, and asked, "This is an unusual name. It is German, no?"

"Yes," I replied. "I was born and raised in Germany."

"Let me tell you something," he went on. "When I was a young man I wanted to become a doctor, and most of all, I wanted to study in Vienna. But my parents did not have enough money to send me there and so I have never seen that city. I have also wanted to study German for all my life. I think it would be great to read in that language in which so much outstanding scientific work has been written."

"Now that's interesting," I told him, "because until my recent retirement, I have spent thirty-five years teaching German."

"Really," he said in astonishment, "you are a German teacher?"

"Yes, I am," I told him, and then he questioned me about where I had taught, and I told him about my interesting career of teaching in the prestigious International Baccalaureate Program – a program with such a rigorous curriculum that students who graduate from it are virtually guaranteed acceptance at most universities. I also told him that my wife and I have been in Vienna many times, and that each of us had been selected to a four-week study fellowship in Vienna through the National Endowment for the Humanities to study Mozart. Vienna had become our favorite city in the world.

The doctor listened attentively, then he handed me a piece of paper and a pen and said, "Would you please let me have your telephone number. That all sounds so fascinating. I might just give you a call." We shook hands and he departed.

Pat returned a minute later and asked me to follow her. She led me to the opposite side of the clinic. After opening one of the dressing rooms for me, she said, "Get undressed in here and put on one of these hospital gowns and make sure the opening is in the back. When you are finished, come out and wait for me inside this room." We stood at the door of a large room in which I saw only the CT table. I went inside the dressing room and put on the hospital gown. I really do not like this apparel. Reason one: I have a hard time tying the strings behind my back, and reason two: it seems that no matter how you tie it, your butt always sticks out.

When I was done, I went out and waited in the scanner room. Pat arrived shortly and noticed that I did not have any socks on (I had come barefoot in sandals). She told me that in the future, I should wear socks. She then asked me to sit on the edge of the table. After she helped me swing my legs on the table and adjust a small cushion under my head, she introduced Brenda. "This is Brenda. She will work with me on these procedures." I lifted my head as much as I could and we greeted each other. Brenda was a pleasant looking brunette.

I laid back on the very flat surface of the table. "If you would please raise your body a little, so we could pull the gown out from under you," I heard Pat say. I lifted a little and the gown was pulled out from under me. "That's great." Now my gown was lifted completely and moved up to somewhere above my belly button. I looked straight up at the ceiling. I could not see the two women at all.

Then Pat said, "Brenda will now shave the treatment area." Again, I could not see anything, but I did feel a razor being pulled several times across the pubic area. Pat continued, "I will now disinfect the tip of your penis. This may feel a little cold at first." I felt something creamy and cool rubbed around the tip. It was not really cold. Pat spoke again, "I will now insert a very short tube into the urethra, so take a deep breath and hold still."

I felt something being inserted very gently into that tiny opening. It did not really hurt, but I definitely felt that something had been stuck into a place where it did not belong. And then I felt the clamp go around the base of my (you know what. I think I have used the p word often enough). I never felt any liquid go inside. Then I was left alone on the table for a time while the scanner did its work. I tried to imagine how I looked there on the table, all by myself in the room, with obviously some kind of tube sticking out of my, yes, you know what. I don't remember how long I laid there, but suddenly the two ladies were back. They stood by the side of the table and I felt each one of them mark an X on the outside of my upper thighs. Then I felt Brenda push gently down several times on the pubic area, about an inch above the (p word) and put an X there, too. Round tapes covered all three X's. After that, it felt as if Pat and Brenda were massaging my legs from just above the knee down to the ankle. I still lay there for a while. Then Pat and Brenda lifted my legs and carefully removed the mold that had been made.

As I lay there, I became aware that a steady stream of cold air was continuously blown across my groin area. What the hell! Without having to look, I knew that maximum shrinkage had occurred down there, and that in full view of the two ladies who did what they had to do in that region. Not exactly the most glorious moment for any man.

Then, everything went very quickly. The gown was pulled back down over me (I had not been aware that anything had been disconnected). Pat and Brenda took my arms and gently helped me sit up. After a few seconds, they swung my legs over the side of the table and I was able to stand up.

"That's it for today," Pat told me. "See you next week for the tattooing."

I changed back into my street clothes, went out to my wife and drove home. All of this had taken about an hour.

At the next session, I felt like a total pro at this thing. Get the ID and key. Find the correct dressing room. Get undressed and put on the gown. Go. When I stepped out of the dressing room I was met by a young man who told me his name was Ted. He motioned me to sit down on one of the chairs outside the radiation room. He also sat down in the chair facing me. He explained what the tattooing procedure was all about. He then led me around a turn to the right and we entered the radiation room. Brenda was waiting for us at the table. I sat down on the table; my legs were swung around and placed into the mold, which was already on the table. I laid back. A slight lift of the buttocks and the gown was moved out from under me. Brenda handed me a plastic ring, about three inches in diameter. I was told to hold this ring with both of my hands resting on my chest. Brenda then pulled up my gown exposing my groin area and Ted placed a sheet strategically right at the base of my (you know what). Then they both tugged at the bed sheet from both sides for adjustment. I was ready. They left the room and then the linear accelerator went into action. The main part of this machine looks like a big donut. It swings around on an arc and comes to rest above the treatment area. There it hovers for a while giving off different kinds of sounds. Then, suddenly, it swings away and another apparatus takes its place. It, too, makes different noises. This one then swings away and an X-ray machine appears in its place. At different intervals, the table gets a slight jolt. I was told that this is an adjustment in the positioning process. It did not take all too long and Brenda and Ted came back into the room.

"Now I will place the tattoos into the marked positions," Ted told me. He went to my right side and I felt a tiny pinch at the exact spot where the X had been marked outside my right thigh. He did the same thing on the left, and then inserted the third tattoo right smack-dab in the middle of the pelvic region, about an inch above the base of my (you know what). He and Brenda rubbed those three areas with some kind of cleansing liquid, but they told me that the previous markings would gradually come off by themselves. That was it.

They helped me off the table. I got my glasses from the shelf where I had left them and was told that, according to the schedule that I had been given before, my actual radiation treatments would begin in two days. So far, so good.

They were ready. I was ready. I did not know what to expect, but I did know that something interesting was about to happen.

Day 1

Dressing room 3. Technicians: Brenda and Donna

I was back in two days, found my ID card and key #3. When I went inside Dressing Room 3, I was in for a surprise. There were no gowns anywhere in sight. Instead, I saw a number of blue squares of cloth neatly stacked up on the hamper where the gowns were last time I was here. I picked one up, and lo and behold, these were actually short pants. They were very large short pants (I guess one size does fit all). When I put them on, I realized that they were very unique pants indeed. The entire front could be flipped open by simply pulling the drawstring, which held the whole thing together. Now this was a breakthrough. I had never liked those hospital gowns, especially those that had to be tied in the back on top and around the waist. It was probably just my own clumsiness, which created my animosity toward those gowns. When I stepped out of the dressing room, I saw a man sitting on one of the chairs outside the radiation room and a female technician, whom I had never seen before, was telling him how great he looked in those pants. Yes, the two of us made quite a lovely pair. Two elderly men in colorful T-shirts, socks, and baggy blue shorts, which would readily fall off with one slight pull of the string. What a fashion statement!

To my surprise, the young lady asked me to come with her first while the other man stayed behind. She introduced herself as we walked toward the back, but I couldn't remember her name. Brenda was there and everything went as before: sit on the table, lift legs to be placed into the mold, hold the ring on your chest, lift

14

buttocks to pull pants down a little, tug of the sheets, pull on the drawstring for treatment exposure. The two ladies left the room and my first radiation treatment began. I had told myself beforehand that I would try to see if there was some kind of pattern to the treatment. Donut first, then the other contraption, then, silence, now a slight buzzing sound, then, a sudden jolt of the table. After a while, I gave up. There was simply too much going on. Let it be – just lie back and relax, I told myself.

Quite honestly, I had no idea how long the treatment lasted. Suddenly, the two technicians were back. They took me by my arms and gently helped me into a sitting position. I gingerly stepped down to the floor. Thank you, ladies. I'll see you tomorrow. When I came home, I told my wife that this was the first time in my life that two women had simultaneously pulled down my pants.

Day 2

Dressing room 3. Technicians: Ted and Brenda

Ted was there to greet me. As we walked into the radiation room, he said, "And how are you today, Mr. Stefan?" Brenda, who had followed us into the room said to him, "He likes to be called by his first name, Helmut."

"Now let me guess," Ted said, "that is a German name, is it not?"

"Yes," I answered, "I was born and raised in Germany."

"Really?" Ted replied. "I don't know any German, but my last name is Sindeldorf."

"That's definitely German," I replied. "The name of my best friend in Germany was Hagendorf, and not far from where I lived there was a town called Wachendorf."

I sat down at the edge of the table. My legs were swung around and placed into the mold, and soon the entire process started over again. This time, I no longer paid any attention to what the machine was doing. Let it do its thing. I tried to relax and lie there as comfortably as possible. I closed my eyes and tried not to think of anything in particular, and for a while I succeeded. All I felt was the cool air blowing across my lower abdomen.

When the machine stopped, I was helped up and was just about ready to leave the room when Ted came to me and said, "You know, there is one thing I really would want to do. Someday, I want to go to Germany."

"Well," I told him, "two years ago my wife and I went to the Oktoberfest in Munich. Now that is something you have to experience. There are twelve huge tents and each one holds about 5,000 people. In the middle of each tent is a brass band, playing continuously. The beer is served in one-liter steins. If you are in the Löwenbrau tent, you only get Löwenbrau beer. If you are in the Spatenbrau tent, then you get their beer. Bratwurst and rotisserie chicken are the main meals. There are also two midways between the tents, lined with roller coasters, carousels, shooting galleries and all kinds of other entertainment. We had the time of our life."

"Wow," he replied, "now that is something I got to do."

Day 3

Dressing room 4. Technicians: Brenda and Donna

I was taken care of today by Brenda and the young lady whose name I did not get last time. Well, her name is Donna. Everything went as usual, but when I had dressed and put my key into the box by the exit, one of the office ladies called me over and led me to a scale.

"I will record your weight today." I stepped on the scale – 162lbs. "The doctor also wants to see you today, so would you please take a seat in Room 1."

I sat down and soon Dr. Sinclair came into the room. We shook hands and he asked me how things were coming along. I told him everything was fine; I had no complaints, and that his technicians were really doing an outstanding job.

"Yes," he said, "that is a great group of people."

And then the subject turned toward erections. "You see," he told me, "it is now as if the prostate is getting a sunburn that is getting worse with each treatment. That does naturally affect a man's ability to get an erection. The good thing, however, is that after the treatments stop, everything gets pretty much back to normal in two to four weeks."

That's good to know, I thought, but I only nodded my head in agreement.

"The reason I wanted to speak with you today is that next week, when we were originally scheduled, I will be out of town. I will see you again after that."

We shook hands, but before I could leave, he continued, "and welcome to the club."

As I drove home that day, I could not get that phrase out of my mind. I repeated to myself, "welcome to the club."

Day 4

Dressing room 4. Technicians: Brenda and Donna

This was the first of my 9:30 AM sessions. I had told the lady in the office that I would appreciate a time in the morning as soon as a slot became available. So here I was at 8:50 a.m., driving along with a full bladder when suddenly Dr. Sinclair's words came to mind, "Welcome to the club."

When I stepped out of the dressing room, I saw that there was one man sitting in front of the radiation room, dressed in the customary blue shorts. He also wore a red T-shirt and black socks, which really did not look very good on him. I said good morning and sat down on the chair next to him. Across from us on the wall was the poster that I had seen now three times. This poster showed the position of the empty bladder and the full bladder. It was clear that the full bladder had moved slightly away from the prostate, thereby giving easier access to it. On top it was the statement, "Why you should have a full bladder for your treatment." Just then a man came around the corner from the radiation room. I looked at him, and then at the poster. The man next to me got up to go into the radiation room. My eyes followed him and then moved back to the poster – and now it hit me. The man who had just come out, the man who now went in, and I, sitting here on this chair, and the hundreds of men who would still come through here, and the thousands of men throughout the world who were undergoing this same treatment. We all belonged to the same club. We were one gigantic brotherhood. We were the FBC. Yes, we were the

20

FULL BLADDER CLUB

Dr. Sinclair had created this thought in me – a club of men, a society, if you will, who had the same experience as all the others, for at least forty-five days, and then went on with their lives, all with great hopes, but how many disappointments?

The Full Bladder Club

I am a member of the Full Bladder Club, at least for a while – and I plan to make the most of it.

Day 5

Dressing room 2. Technicians: Donna and Ted

When I picked up my key today, I noticed that I was assigned dressing room 2. I remembered that during the first four visits, I had been in room 3 two times and in room 4 also two times. This made me think. There are four dressing rooms outside of the radiation room. I will use them for a total of 45 times. Now, I am not a good mathematician, but according to the law of averages, I should have used each room somewhere around ten or eleven times by the time my treatment is over. And yet, I also learned that if a coin lands on heads ten times in a row, there is no guarantee that the next time it will land on tails. The chance at each toss is fifty-fifty. This all makes sense. Well, from now on, I will record which dressing room I use at each visit, and when it's all over, we will see how this law of averages worked out.

Day 6

Dressing room 3. Technicians: Ted and Brenda

As I lay on the table today, with the machine going through its circular motions, and having read again and again, when the machine stopped at a specific place, "This is the X-ray machine. It's not in use during radiation treatment," I came to the conclusion that I had to spend this time here on the table in a more constructive and productive manner. Sure, it was so easy to fall into a semi-trance or just let one's mind wander aimlessly. It's not that this would be a waste of time (I certainly could afford these ten minutes) but this was a special circumstance, something that not everyone experiences, and I wanted to see what I could come up with during this duration of time which had been forced on me. (I know, I know, I agreed to this treatment method). No matter how I looked at it, these ten minutes were a special period of time in my life. I decided that for each session I would either have a topic ready (relive the places we have traveled to; go back to my childhood years as a refugee in Germany; my years of teaching; my courtship and marriage to the most wonderful woman in the world; music, yes music, the art form that has given me so much; recent news headlines, etc., etc., the number of topics is absolutely inexhaustible).

Day 7

Dressing room 3. Technicians: Ted and Donna

The topic I had chosen for today was "jokes." That did not happen by chance. You see, last night we had dinner with Carl and Veronica. They are wonderful people and Carl possesses that great trait to tell jokes, which I don't have, and for which I admire him and all the people who possess it. Almost every time we meet, Carl greets me with, "Have you heard about the man who was walking down the street with his dog...?" Then comes the pause, and I either reply, "No, I haven't," or I just shrug my shoulders and wait. And then comes the joke. It is always funny and I know that he has a lot more of them in store for me, and I will hear some of them as the evening progresses. My father was a great teller of jokes, too, and although in his older years, (he lived to be 91) he told some of the jokes again and again, they were still funny, because there was always a slight variation in the way he told them, that still made listening to him a great experience. The fact that we all knew what the punch line would be made absolutely no difference.

Well, I did not inherit that gift. When I hear a joke that I really like, I make it a special point to remember it. But it has happened time and time again that I could not, no matter how hard I tried, to remember the joke, or if I did remember it, I would botch it up so badly that it really wasn't very funny by the time I got through telling it. Sometimes I would only remember the punch line, but what was the beginning of the joke?

24

Now, I do remember several jokes. This one I remember because I first told it at a very special occasion in my life. It was at our fortieth wedding anniversary celebration with family and friends. This is a joke that was either told by Henny Youngman or by Red Skelton. There seems to be some disagreement among my friends. Here's the joke:

> *A couple is celebrating their fiftieth wedding anniversary. As they sit at the head table and watch their guests dance and have a good time, a young man approaches them and says, "What is the secret behind your long and happy marriage?"*
> *The old man looks at him and replies, "My wife and I go out to a romantic dinner twice a week – soft music, candlelight, dancing, good food, champagne – she goes on Tuesdays and I go on Fridays."*

Day 8

Dressing room 3. Technicians: Ted and Brenda

When today's session was over and I had gotten off the table, I said to Brenda, "It's true that everything is relative. Today's session just seemed shorter than the previous ones." Brenda then told me that I was not the first person to say this. It seems that the time on the table appears to get shorter to the patient as the number of treatments increases. "There is something else I just realized." I went on, "All the time I thought that the ceiling lights went on and off during the treatment, but now I just noticed that some of the lights get blocked off when the machine goes through its rotary motion." Then I turned to Ted and asked, "Just out of curiosity, what is the distance between the various parts of the machine and my body during treatment?" Ted showed me where the table would be and where the machine would be during an actual treatment session. "I would say the distance is about 18 inches," he replied. I told both of them that I was keeping a daily journal and that I would share it with them when I was finished. They both seemed delighted by the idea and told me that they would gladly cooperate with me in any way they possibly could to contribute to my experience. Those two are absolutely super!

Day 9

Dressing room 3. Technicians: Ted and Donna

As soon as I walked into the waiting area, I knew something was wrong. There was one man sitting here, I had seen him before, and before I could say anything, he said, "Yup, they're back." He sat there in a hospital gown and again with black socks on. "Oh, no," I said. "This is cause for a revolution." The man actually looked serious as he replied, "Yeah, I don't like these damned things either." So I went to Room 3 and clumsily tied the strings together. Whoever invented this garment should be shot.

When I walked into the radiation room, I noticed for the first time how many sets of leg molds were lined up along the walls. If they used all of these molds in one day, that had to come to quite some number.

Today I got a pleasant surprise (not the hospital gowns). Ted asked me whether I would like to look at the monitors, which the technicians viewed during treatment. I was absolutely delighted. Donna pulled up my chart and now I could see my pelvis and the fiducial markers that had been implanted in my prostate. She then showed me how these three markers are lined up inside three circles that are on the diagram of my pelvic region. When the three markers are inside the circles, the alignment is complete and the treatment can begin.

When I asked whether the linear accelerator beams the radiation only from above and the sides (I had observed only a 180 degree movement of the Gantry which moved across the body), Ted explained, "No, radiation occurs from all sides, that is, 360 degrees. However, the machine does not go around and around. It moves back and forth. The duration and amount of radiation is the same for every patient. There are no different degrees of treatment between patients."

That was something I had not expected. I thought there were different levels of the disease and therefore different levels of treatment. Well, that shows once again that there is always something new to learn.

Day 10

Dressing room 1. Technicians: Ted and Donna

Well now, here is something new. This was the first time that I was assigned to dressing room 1. On the walls were two black and white photographs. The larger one showed Big Ben in London and the smaller one showed the Dome of Sacre Coeur sticking out from between various shaped roofs in Paris. To think of it, there also was a black and white photograph in dressing room 3, also a cityscape, but I can't remember it. I will pay more attention to the decorations inside the different dressing rooms and try to learn if some interior decorator had tried to establish some sort of theme that was related to the purpose of these rooms. Somehow I doubt that. And those damned hospital gowns were still there.

Day 11

Dressing room 4. Technicians: Ted and Donna

Here I am back again in dressing room 4. There are no pictures on the walls. This is a slightly larger room than the others, and there is a door, which leads to a washroom. This, I find rather amusing, for on the door is a sign that states, "STOP – your treatment requires a full bladder" – so much for the utility of the washroom.

Right from the beginning, I had been told that when the patient lies on the table, he can talk to the technicians in the other room, and they can talk to him. So, before I laid down on the table, I asked Donna and Ted whether today they couldn't say a few words to me through the intercom, because I was interested to hear what their voices would sound like under the buzzing accelerator and with them being in the other room about twenty feet away. Donna said that Ted could sing me a song, but Ted protested and claimed that I would probably jump off the table if he began to sing. Once they left the room, I waited for a voice, and within a few seconds, I heard Donna say, "OK, you're in position now." I replied, "All right, go ahead." Then I heard her voice again, very distinctly and gently say, "I will now begin your treatment." And the machine began its continuous back and forth movement.

Day 12

Dressing room 3. Technicians: Ted and Brenda

As I sat by myself in the waiting area waiting to be called in for treatment, I finally realized what this entire experience has been lacking – the interaction with other men who were going through the same thing as I was. In a way, this was a compliment to the way the treatments were scheduled and then efficiently carried out. If you arrived on time, you should be in the radiation room within minutes, and when you left, the next patient would be ready to go in. So far, I never had to wait for more than a few minutes. This was good, because this clockwork treatment made it possible for each of us to plan our day around each session. And yet, I wished that perhaps one day there would be at least one man, or two, or even three, waiting to be treated. (Not more, there are only four chairs available). I think it would be interesting to talk to these men, to find out how many sessions they have already had. Were they all family men with supportive families behind them, like me, or was there perhaps a widower without children (or with children who had moved away) who had to face this all by himself? Were they suffering from other ailments and was this the straw that broke the camel's back? What had they experienced in life and did they, like me, never expect to wind up here, bare-butted in a hospital gown, just wearing socks and a T-shirt? How optimistic were they that everything would be all right or had maybe one or the other thrown in the towel and was ready and willing to die? Were they still working, or were they retired, and what did they do for a living? When I saw a man come out of the radiation room, or when I saw the next man waiting to go in after me, I could not tell anything about them – professor or truck driver? Dentist, store clerk or mechanic? There was always a quick smile, a nod of the head, and a hurried "hi" between us. Here, in the patient waiting room, we were all the same – all afflicted with the same disease, all undergoing the same treatment. What was everyone thinking? I don't know. That is what made us all unique. And yet, as we shuffled along in our clumsily tied gowns and with our different colored socks, we had one thing in common. We were all FBC's – members of the FULL BLADDER CLUB.

Day 13

Dressing room 4. Technicians: Ted and Donna

Today is one of those dark, blustery pre-autumn days that I remember all too well from my childhood in Germany. We did not live very far from the North Sea in the north and the English Channel in the west – and those cold wet winds would continue for days on end. But this weather also reminds me of something that the three of us, my friends Heiner, Peter and I would do at this time of year. We all lived in a village consisting of five farms that were fairly close together. Scattered around the larger town in which we went to school, there were several other such villages. Now, I don't remember how all of this started, but this had become a tradition by the time I was ten years old.

Not far from our village was a pond hidden in the woods. Each year, the boys from the various villages vied as to who would be the first, after the winter had passed, to go skinny-dipping in the pond; and in the late fall, who would be the last to do the same thing before winter arrived. The contest was that you had to be completely immersed in the water to make it count. So on just a day like this one, the three of us would go down to the pond, quickly undress, wade waist deep into the pond and then a quick dip – total immersion – and then out as quickly as possible. We did not have any towels with us and so we jumped around like wild monkeys to get at least a little dry before putting our clothes back on. Why did we have to do this butt naked? Because our mothers had long ago put our swimming trunks away somewhere, and, of course, mom and especially dad, were not supposed to know about this.

The three of us always won this contest (for nothing but bragging rights). This was maybe because we lived closest to the pond, or maybe because we were just the biggest idiots. That we could have become seriously sick from these crazy escapades, well, that thought never entered our silly little heads.

Day 14

Dressing room 1. Technicians: Ted and Donna

I have not noticed this before, but by the elevator, next to the sign that is mounted on a metal stand, there is another sign that also says Center for Prostate Cancer. This elevator only goes down, and the thought has occurred to me that if above the elevator door one could read that most frightful of all messages, "Abandon all hope ye who enter herein," then one could easily imagine that one was about to enter the first circle of Dante's *Inferno*. It is also ironic that above the LL button, there is a small plate attached to the elevator wall that says Press Button Hard. So, if you just touch the button, like I did for the first time, the elevator doesn't go anywhere. You have to definitely assert that you want to go down there. On the way down to the *Inferno*, the eternally doomed have no choice; here, we push the button hard to descend to the lower level, because we know we are not doomed – that down there, we will not be punished (well, a little bit) and that we will come up again healthier than we were before.

Day 15

Dressing room 3. Technicians: Brenda and Donna

Today was a special day for three reasons: 1) the pants were back in the dressing rooms. When I entered the waiting area the man sitting in one of the four chairs wearing the blue pants and a green T-shirt gave me a thumbs up and said, "Hallelujah." I returned the sign and said to myself, "Amen." 2) My wife came along today and brought her camera with her. This had been pre-planned, because when I told the staff that I was writing a journal about this whole experience, and that I would appreciate pictures of the entire team and, if possible, some pictures of me on the table, they had readily agreed to participate and cooperate in every way. They are just the most fantastic group of people you will ever want to meet. So here I am now on the table with Brenda and Donna by my side. Another picture shows my upper thigh and the crossed lines meeting exactly over the tattoo, which had been placed there before the treatments began. Then there is a picture of Donna, Brenda, Pat, Ted and me, all with big smiles on our faces, complete with me in my big, blue shorts. On the way out, my wife and I stopped in the main office were we took a picture of Megan, the receptionist, Jan the nurse, and me. Unfortunately, Tina, the medical assistant, was not there that day. All of these pictures will play a cherished role when someday I will think back to this unique time in my life. 3) Today I received my fifteenth treatment. That means that I am one-third through with the program. On the one hand, it seems that this has been a long journey everything has become so routine and it is hard for me to recall when it all started. On the other hand, however, it is hard to fathom that three weeks have already gone by. Soon I will reach the half-way-point and then I will head for the finish line. I wonder how I will feel physically and mentally when all of this is over. If things continue the way they are right now, I will be more than pleased. But more importantly, will a final stop have been made to this dreadful disease, which just wants to grow and grow and has put so many men, sometimes so prematurely, into the grave?

Day 16

Dressing room 4. Technicians: Ted and Brenda

Today is Friday and it is one of those glorious days that we treasure so much here in the Midwest. It is a precursor of Indian summer weather that we look forward to all year. And the good news is that this splendid weather is to continue throughout the weekend and well into the next week.

But that's not all the good news today. As I came out of the radiation room, I saw the linen man carry in an armful of those detestable hospital gowns. "Will we ever get our pants back again?" I asked him. "Yes, they'll be here again next Tuesday," he replied, as he put down the stack of gowns. Well, that made my day and the entire weekend. Being in such good spirits, I think this is the right time to tell the second of my four jokes.

> *An old man, obviously in very bad physical shape, comes to a doctor's office and says, "Doc, could you please prescribe some of them Viagra pills for me?" The doctor looks him over and says, "My dear man, given your age and physical condition, do you really still have to be involved with women?" The old man gives the doctor a stern look and says, "Women? Who said anything about women? I just don't want to pee on my shoes all the time anymore!"*

Day 17

Dressing room 3. Technicians: Ted and Donna

Two sessions ago I stated that the elevator down to the Center for Prostate Cancer reminded me of going down to the first circle of Dante's *Inferno*. That, of course, was a joke. When the elevator door opens, one floor below, the first thing that you see is an aquarium (hardly the first thing that you will see upon entering the first circle of hell, although that is supposed to be the nicest one). The aquarium is quite large, I would say that it is five feet wide, two feet high, and one foot deep. The water is very clear and there are interesting plants and objects in it. There are also six very colorful, differently sized fish swimming serenely back and forth. Above the tank is a big basket of artificial flowers, and on both sides of these flowers are numerous stuffed animals – all some sort of sea creatures. They would be wonderful playthings for little children, but little children don't come down here. Above all of this are very bright lights, which really don't do those flowers any good. There also is a flat screen TV mounted on a wall, and a door that leads to a washroom. There are two pictures on the wall depicting snails or some other sea animals. There are twelve chairs in this room and another door with a sign on it, which says Escorted Access Only. And I seriously doubt that in the *Inferno* there is a smiling lady who does not push you, but rather politely asks you to follow her.

Day 18

Dressing room 2. Technicians: Ted and Brenda

The side effects of the radiation treatment have definitely made themselves known. I got up three times to urinate last night, and it was a slow and almost painful process before the first trickle appeared. A mild burning sensation has occurred, as the flow got stronger. So far, this was still tolerable, but I remembered Dr. Sinclair's words about the sunburn that gets worse and worse until one can finally withdraw into the cool and soothing shade. But that is still a long way off.

This experience once again brought back some childhood memories. I remember how the same two friends and I would go behind the farmer's barn, stand next to each other and pull down our pants (our pants did not have zippers). Then we would see who could pee the highest against the barn wall. In the winter, when there was snow on the ground, we simply went for distance. Oh well, boys will be boys!

Day 19

Dressing room 4. Technicians: Ted and Donna

When Ted and I came out of the radiation room today, we found Brenda, Donna and Pat, the chief therapist, gathered around the monitors, which are in a separate room outside of the radiation room. As always, they were very friendly and cheerful. I received the same friendly and cheerful good-byes from the three ladies who work in the main office. On my way home, I thought to myself, 'That Ted is sure one hell of a lucky guy. All day long he's in the company of some really wonderful and charming women.' To be sure, I had some very pleasant female colleagues in my thirty-five year teaching career, but I was never so totally surrounded by them as Ted obviously is.

But then, another thought occurred to me. All day long, Ted is also involved with one geezer after another, all of them in their ill-fitting gowns or pants, black socks or not, lying there semi-exposed on the table, trying to control their bladders – all of this is obviously not a very pretty sight.

Oh well, I guess there are two sides to every story.

Day 20

Dressing room 4. Technicians: Ted and Brenda

After today's radiation session, I had my weekly meeting with Dr. Sinclair. He asked me how I was coming along, and I told him that the side effects that I had been told about and, which I had also read about, were definitely making themselves felt. "How so?" he asked. I told him about the two or three nightly trips to the bathroom, the difficulty in getting the first trickle to appear, and the not exactly pleasant feeling once the urine actually begins to flow hesitantly. "Any burning sensations?" he asked me. I told him that I would be hesitant to use the word 'burning,' but it sure wasn't the same as before. "You are displaying the classic symptoms that accompany this treatment," he told me. "Why don't you try taking three ibuprofens before you go to sleep. That might help with the frequency problem." I told him that I would and that we would discuss this next week. Dr. Sinclair agreed, we shook hands, and I left the office.

Once I entered the main office area, Jan, the nurse, intercepted me. She told me that she would take me to Petra, the Clinical Dietitian, who was scheduled to meet with me today.

I was led into an office back on the side of the building where the radiation room is located. Petra got up from behind her desk and greeted me most cordially. There was something very pleasant about her entire demeanor, and I liked her immediately.

We went over the same questions: frequency of urination, burning, lighter stool, etc. She addressed each problem in a very professional manner. She also produced several sheets of paper with titles like Eating Right for Good Health; Nutrition and Physical Activity Goals; Constipation; Diarrhea, Gas/Flatulence; Urinary Tract Irritants; Heart-Healthy Eating Nutrition Therapy; Ways to Reduce Sodium. Furthermore, all of this was broken down into food groups – milk, meat and other protein foods, fruits and vegetables, grains. This was then divided up into foods recommended and foods not recommended. Petra then gave a very succinct explanation why this was recommended over that, and why drinking a lot of water throughout the day was beneficial, etc., etc. She was, of course, very proficient, but one could sense that the patient's well being seriously mattered to her. As I was leaving, she told me not to hesitate to stop in her office if I had any concerns. I promised her I would do that should the need arise.

Day 21

Dressing room 1. Technicians: Donna and Brenda

The autumnal solstice took place last night at 9:29 p.m.; fall has arrived. The days will become shorter and the nights proportionally longer. Where has the summer gone? I remember that when I was a child, I could not wait for Christmas to come. The time seemed so long until we went out and cut down our Christmas tree, decorated it with real candles, tinsel and walnuts that were painted silver or gold and hung from colorful ribbons. This was in the harsh post World War II years in utterly defeated and destroyed Germany. The gifts for my brother and me usually consisted of hand knitted mittens or scarves that my mother and grandmother had worked on in the little free time that they had. We were ecstatic if there was a rubber ball among the gifts. That was something very special. And yet, I longed for the days of Christmas, and they always seemed so far away.

And now another season has passed. Yes, it is true what the old people had said (and which I never believed) time just moves along faster when you get older. The first touches of red, yellow and gold are visible in the trees. Soon they will be gone, too. And then comes that long quiet time of looking out the window, watching the snow fall gently, and longing for the next spring; new light, colors and life. How many more times will I experience this joy, this exhilarating feeling, granted, being old, but still being there among all of that which is fresh, young and jubilant? How many more times?

44

Day 22

Dressing room 2. Technicians: Brenda and Donna

Today I had to wait for a few minutes because the man ahead of me was still being treated. I looked around for something to read. I had already perused the magazines that are on a low table, which has two chairs on the left, and two chairs on the right of it. But there is another small table underneath the infamous, "Why You Need a Full Bladder" poster. I went over to it and found two copies of the Wall Street Journal and one copy of Modern Photography. And next to that little table hangs a small sign, which reads, "Do not take magazines into washroom."

Now I know that there are many clinics throughout the country where men go to make a "donation." It is my understanding that at these clinics, magazines (picture magazines) are provided for these "donors" just in case they have a hard time rising to the occasion. In other words, these magazines are to help them reach that level of concentration that is needed to get the job done.

To top it all off, next to the Wall Street Journal and Modern Photography (not exactly inspirational in my book) there stands a bottle of hand lotion and a box of Kleenex.

Now, you may say that I am just a dirty old man. Well, that's quite all right with me, because my wife has told me on more than one occasion that this is one of the reasons why she loves me – and that is all that really matters to me.

Day 23

Dressing room 2. Technicians: Brenda and Donna

Today I have reached the half way point in my treatments. Where has the time gone? To be sure, the treatments have become routine, but my daily encounter with the office staff and my wonderful technicians make every day a unique experience.

I also feel quite good. The side effects of the treatment have not become worse; as a matter of fact, they have improved. The three ibuprofens I take before going to bed have decreased the frequency of the nightly visits to the bathroom; everything flows more readily and easily and I really feel good all over. When I see Dr. Sinclair next week, I will ask him whether my stomach pains (always at night) and that bloated feeling are side effects of the treatment. But maybe they will be gone by then. I would be very pleased if things stayed the way they are right now until the end of the treatment period. Anyway: twenty-three down, twenty-two to go. I think I'll make it just fine!

Day 24

Dressing room 2. Technicians: Ted and Brenda

On the way to the clinic this morning, I heard the final few minutes of Schubert's 8th Symphony, the Unfinished. This is one of my all time favorite pieces of classical music – and I'll tell you why: First of all, it is simply one of the most beautiful compositions ever written (I will not accept any arguments about this). And secondly, it is this composition that opened the wonderful world of classical music for me.

This is how it happened: I think I must have been a junior in high school, when one afternoon my friend Pete dropped by at the house and showed me the 33 rpm record he had just bought at the local supermarket for 99 cents. On the one side it had Beethoven's 5th Symphony, and on the other side, Schubert's 8th Symphony. Since we had already heard the Beethoven piece in our music class, we decided to listen to the Schubert composition. Pete told me that the record was a gift for his father who loved classical music, but that their record player at home was broken.

The music began, and a whole new world opened for me. The piece starts with the violins playing agitated eighth notes bouncing up and down, up and down. Then, an oboe enters and plays a plaintive melody, which is interrupted by sudden loud chords. The violins continue in the bouncing rhythm, the oboe enters again, loud chords, but then, unexpectedly, a French horn holds a long, very long note, and then the violins put down a subdued foundation with their syncopated rhythm, and now finally comes what I consider to be one of the greatest moments in musical history: the cellos enter with perhaps the most beautiful melody ever conceived by the mind of man (a genius, in this case). Soon the other strings enter and sweep away with the original theme, and it all becomes simply one of the most glorious moments in the history of music.

"If this is classical music," I thought to myself, "then I want more of it." And more of it I got. I listened to the classical station on the radio; I bought cheap records, (CD's were still some time away) and Pete and I went to the free outdoor summer concerts presented by our city's superb symphony orchestra. I soon realized that besides Schubert, Mozart and Beethoven had become my favorites, and they still are to this very day.

The great Russian composer Peter Ilyitch Tchaikovsky was once asked whether Schubert's music, with its long themes and many repeats, doesn't put him to sleep? "Yes, it does," the famous composer replied, "but when I wake up, it seems like I've been in heaven."

Day 25

Dressing room 3. Technicians: Brenda and Donna

I am so glad that they have a sense of humor in this place. There is a sign under the television set in the waiting area outside of the radiation room. This is what it says:

> *Everyone here wants to help you.*
>
> *You have to wear the gown for nine weeks,*
> *Smile as you walk around hiding your*
> *cheeks.*
>
> *The therapists deal with this every day,*
> *All they ask is that you do as they say.*
>
> *NO TENSE BUTTS she said,*
> *You comply hoping your face doesn't turn*
> *red.*
>
> *You pray as you walk through the door,*
> *Please don't let me piddle on the floor.*

Honestly, you couldn't make this stuff up!

Day 26

Dressing room 1. Technicians: Ted and Brenda

As I walked into the treatment area waiting room I saw that something had certainly changed – and there was Donna with a big poster of a monster in her hand, which she was just about to tape on the door of dressing room 3. I hadn't even thought about Halloween, but the crew down here obviously did not forget. My dressing room had a "Do not Enter" on it with a doorknocker, which you supposedly had to use before you could enter. On one wall was a big poster of a coffin with some kind of ghoul ready to come out of it. Even when I went around the corner to enter the treatment room, there was a sign on it that said, "Do not Enter." But enter I did.

I questioned Donna whether the room where we receive our treatment is actually called the radiation room. She said that it could be called that, but that it is actually the "vault." That makes sense. There is a door that leads into this room, and this door is at least eight inches thick. I was also told that the linear accelerator, which delivers the radiation, does not go on unless the door is closed. I can easily imagine that this multi-million dollar machine needs to be safely locked up when not in use.

I also asked Donna if she, Brenda and Ted are actually called technicians. "No." she replied, "We are called therapists." Now that is something I should have figured out for myself, because if Pat is the chief therapist, then the people she works with had to be therapists.

Okay, I'll be the first to admit that sometimes the old noodle just doesn't work that well anymore (double entendre intended).

Day 27

Dressing room 3. Therapists: Donna and Brenda

I had to see Dr. Sinclair after today's session. First, I was weighed, and I was happy to learn that I had lost three pounds since the therapy began. This was not due to the radiation treatment, but rather because before I began with the treatment, I told myself that I would like to lose nine pounds during the nine week period – one pound a week. That seemed a reasonable thing to do, since I could definitely afford to shed a few pounds. So, I watched myself a little more than usual. Instead of 2% milk, we switched to 1% (as the nutritionist suggested). Of course, avoid heavy and greasy foods, portion control, etc. The problem is that I have a healthy appetite (the treatment up to now has not made an impact). On the plus side, I have a wife who is a tremendous cook, who not only prepares delicious meals, but also knows how to make them healthy and nourishing.

Dr. Sinclair was his usual cheerful self as he asked me how I was coming along. I told him that lately peeing had become quite difficult (yes, I said peeing, because I am tired of saying urinating when everyone knows what it really means). I also told him that the burning sensation was not too bad, but it definitely did not feel normal. Dr. Sinclair told me that there was medication available to help with the flow problem, but first he would like me to try a more conservative approach (before adding more medication). "Take the three ibuprofens twice a day, once before bedtime and once in the afternoon, and let me know if that helps." I said that I would do this. Then I told him about my stomach problems – how at different times of the day, and even at night, I would suddenly get a burning sensation that made it seem as if my entire abdomen was aflame. I explained to him that Maalox helped, or that at other times, after a flare up, I would let a couple of Tums dissolve in my mouth and that helped, too. But it simply has not gone away like it has at other times when this has occurred. Dr. Sinclair advised me not to wait for an attack to happen, but to take a few spoonful of Maalox, or something like it, after every meal. "Let's see how that works out for now. Come and see me tomorrow if nothing has changed." Well, let's see what happens.

Day 28

Dressing room 1. Therapists: Brenda and Donna

I guess in one respect we are all pretty much alike: as long as something doesn't really bother us, we don't pay any attention to it. That certainly was the case with me. Of course, I knew that I had a prostate gland inside of me, and I knew pretty much where it was supposed to be. After all, my doctor had performed the digital prostate examination on me often enough; I knew about the PSA number, and I knew that it was the most common form of cancer in men, after skin cancer. But now, that I had the disease, I decided to take a closer look at the whole thing. And so I did what probably most people would do, I went to the Internet and typed in the word "prostate" and bingo, there it was. I clicked on the first entry and immediately had a picture in front of me, a side-view cross section of a man's body from the bladder downwards. The caption read, "The prostate is a walnut-sized gland located between the bladder and the penis. The prostate is just in front of the rectum. The urethra runs through the center of the prostate, from the bladder to the penis, letting urine flow out of the body. The prostate secretes fluid that nourishes and protects sperm. During ejaculation, the prostate squeezes this fluid into the urethra, and it's expelled with sperm as semen."

If there is one good side to this disease, it is that it strikes mostly older men who have already fathered their children. Therefore, walnut-sized gland, I thank you for holding out and staying healthy up until now. Because you did your job when it counted the most, my wife and I are the happy parents of two of the most wonderful kids on earth.

Day 29

Dressing room 4. Therapists: Donna and Brenda

The Urological Clinic and the Center for Prostate Cancer are housed in a quite attractive building. It is constructed of yellow brick and has a most symmetrical form. The center of the building is two stories tall. It is flanked on each side by a wing, which in turn, is then flanked again, slightly recessed, by yet another wing. The roofs of the two wings were low slung and become lower as they spread away from the center. The windows in the center and in the first wings are vertical; they become horizontal in the end wings, which are the lowest. Approximately two inches inside the window frame, there is a one-inch silver strip, which follows the contours of the window. All of this is very reminiscent of the Prairie School buildings that were designed by Frank Lloyd Wright. I am sure that the architect who designed this building had Frank Lloyd Wright in mind when he drew up the plans for this structure. And a good idea that was, too. The way the building is set back from the street and surrounded by trees, it is a welcome sight from those huge structures that one sees everywhere; buildings that house dozens of doctor offices, drug stores, coffee shops, etc. I, for one, find this building aesthetically very pleasing.

Day 30

Dressing room 3. Therapists: Ted and Donna

It finally happened today – the way I knew it would eventually happen. On the way to the clinic, they finally played Mozart on the classical music station to which my car radio is always set. Not just any Mozart piece, mind you, but the overture to the Marriage of Figaro. Here we hear Mozart at his bubbling, boisterous, life-affirming best. As I stated before, ever since my high school years, I have been a fan of classical music, and as the years progressed, Mozart gradually became my favorite of all the great composers who have blessed us with their inspired creations. To be sure, I stand in awe before the majesty of J. S. Bach's immortal creations. And there is Beethoven, who seizes the listener and pulls him along into his creative world of will and imagination. There are so many others whose works I greatly admire and appreciate, but I always come back to Mozart. It is not easy to explain why that is so; there is just something in his music that draws you in – there is charm and wit and flights of fancy that are just irresistible – and he makes it sound all so easy. Someone once said that Mozart simply took down dictation directly from God. Mozart himself insisted that he worked hard to acquire the technical skill necessary to produce one masterpiece after another.

When we think of Mozart, we think first of all of that ultimate child prodigy. He learned the fundamentals of violin playing while watching his father and his friends play string quartets. He repeated phrases on the piano after one hearing – and this at the age of five or six. At the age of eleven, he was commissioned to write an opera. As he and his family traveled through Europe, they were invited to play before kings and queens of most of the European royal houses. Everywhere where he and his sister Maria Anna, affectionally called "Nannerl," appeared (she was five years older and also a musical genius), they created a sensation. One story tells of when little Wolfgang slipped on the shiny parquet floor at Empress Maria Theresia's Schönbrunn Palace, one of her many daughters went to the wunderkind and helped him to get back on his feet. He said, "Thank you. One day I will marry you." That, of course, caused some amusement at the royal court. The little princess who helped him up was none other than Marie Antoinette, and her fate was as tragic as Wolfgang's would eventually be.

One day, while I was grading papers in my classroom, the French teacher from the next room came to me and handed me a brochure. It was a pamphlet from the National Endowment for the Humanities, which advertised summer enrichment courses for American teachers. My fellow teacher had circled the course offering titled, "Mozart, the Man, his Music and his Vienna." They were looking for fifteen teachers from across the United States to participate in this program. I applied, and much to my amazement, I was chosen to be part of this select group. My wife came along, and while I attended the daily sessions in the morning, she was free to enjoy the most wonderful city in the world – Vienna.

Seven years later, my wife was chosen to participate in a similar seminar, "Mozart and his World." Now I had the mornings free to explore every part of Vienna. Each seminar lasted four weeks, and those were some of the happiest days we spent in our lives.

Since then, I have greatly expanded my musical library, mostly with the works by Mozart – now available on CD's. I have also read everything on Mozart I could get my hands on. I devoured it all, but I was amazed at how different scholars came to different conclusions about his great man's life and works.

In 1984, the film Amadeus was released at the movies, then on television and later on DVD. This film was extremely popular, and I, too, enjoyed it very much. It focuses mainly on the last ten years of Mozart's life. It is lively and entertaining, and all of the music is by the master himself – a truly enjoyable movie.

But there is one problem: the movie consists of more fiction than fact. Scene after scene shows Mozart doing things that he never did; people say and do things to him that are not documented anywhere, and the timing of some events is just plain wrong. The movie is still very enjoyable, if one takes this biographical sketch with a grain of salt.

I was asked by a number of people, who know my love for Mozart, what I thought of the film, and I gave them my opinion. This was followed by invitations from reading groups, libraries and coffee houses to talk about my thoughts on Mozart and the movie. And so, I gave numerous talks on the subject, which I titled, "The Mozart Myths." I am happy to say that my talks were well attended and well received.

I love Mozart primarily for his music, but also for the man he was. He was a genius, of course, but also a most down to earth man. He mingled with kings and queens, (he was even knighted by Pope Clement XIV, who praised his music with "the sweetest sound of cymbals"), but he stayed true to his roots. He loved to bowl, dance and shoot air guns at targets. He wrote a funeral cantata when his pet bird died. He loved to joke around, drink a little too much at times, and loved the attention he got from attractive women. His letters, of which hundreds have survived, are filled with acute observations and a sometimes scatological sense of humor that would certainly offend many of the more sensitive readers.

Mozart is the only composer who excelled in all forms of composition of his day. He was a master in writing sonatas, concertos, operas, oratories, symphonies, masses, dance music, requiems – everything he did musically was absolutely astounding.

His mischievous nature and over-bubbling spirit is best demonstrated in a canon in six voices. It is a serious and complex work, and it may hold the listener spellbound by the virtuosity of its construction, until one realizes, that the German word phrases, repeated over and over again in the most imaginative way, are best translated in English by the words, "You can kiss my ass."

Wolfgang Amadeus Mozart died at the age of thirty-five. He was buried in an unmarked grave in St. Marx Cemetery in Vienna. Much later, a statue was erected in the area where his burial place was suspected to be. This memorial shows a broken pillar against which leans a grieving, weeping angel, holding an extinguished torch down to the ground.

My eyes were filled with tears when I stood there some years ago, and every time I look at the picture of this cemetery marker, I am filled with deep melancholy.

But we cannot end our thoughts of Mozart on a sad note. Here is an anecdote told about him: A young man comes to see Mozart and asks, "Master, I am a student of music, and I now want to write a symphony. What advice do you have for me?" Mozart answers: "My dear friend, you are still so young, and writing a symphony is quite a serious and demanding undertaking." "But," replies the young man impatiently, "I heard that you were much

younger than I am when you wrote your first symphony."
"That is true," Mozart responds, "but I didn't ask anyone
how to do it."

Day 31

Dressing room 4. Therapists: Ted and Donna

As I'm lying on the table today, my thoughts go back to music and to how much joy it has brought me in my life. My question is: with today's technology, wouldn't it be easy to pipe music into the vault while the treatment is going on? I envision the whole thing this way: outside the vault there is a touch screen which lists the various kinds of music – country, jazz, blues, swing, hip-hop, classical, etc. The patient chooses one of these categories. Then the artist's name appears, and the patient can select his favorite piece. For myself, I choose classical; then Mozart; then, for example, Piano Concerto No. 21 in C major. I go into the vault, the therapists put me into the proper position, and when they leave and the massive door closes behind them, the music begins. Oh, yes, that glorious music fills the room. I close my eyes and let myself be swept away by the joyful, jubilant introduction. I wait for the piano to enter and repeat the exposition and begin its brilliant variations. Ah, yes, this is the way to do it. Why can't they do it? Time would go by so quickly and so pleasantly.

But the more I think about it, the more doubtful I become that all of this would work – and my doubts were just set off by the word 'quickly.' You see, there is one thing that I cannot stand, that I absolutely abhor – and that is not being able to hear a piece of music to the end, or at least, up to the place where some kind of logical break occurs, like at the end of a movement. More than once have I driven around our block at least ten times just to be able to hear the end of a favorite piece of music. And so, I can envision the following scenario: The treatment has ended and the therapists have reentered the vault. They want to remove my leg molds and help me off the table. But I absolutely refuse – the music is still playing, the climax is about to take place. But they want me off the table. I resist. At first they try gently, but as I refuse to budge, they pull me forcefully. I can see me falling to the floor and taking one of the ladies down with me. By now, my pants are down around my ankles (they hadn't been tied up yet). The other therapist tries to pull me away, but I hold on to the metal rack that stands along the left wall. The whole thing comes tumbling down and smashes into the multi-million dollar linear accelerator. Shrieks of horror – flashing warning lights. By now the vault is filled with people and eventually they, of course, subdue me. I am taken back to my dressing room where I gradually calm down and get dressed. I sneak out as quickly as I can and drive home with my hands shaking on the steering wheel; my heart beating as if it wants to get out of my chest.

And that's not the end of it. I still have to go back there tomorrow; after all, I need to get fourteen more treatments. I'm not sure that I will be able to withstand the disdainful looks that I am bound to get. No more cheerful hellos and goodbyes. Everything will be changed, all due to my fanaticism about music.

And so, maybe it is better to lie there in silence and hear the grinding, the whizzing and the clicking noises of the machine. Sounds that put me in a semi-stupor, that make my mind wander off into unknown realms, and maybe, just maybe, then I will come up with another crazy story just like this one.

Day 32

Dressing room 1. Therapists: Brenda and Donna

Today is a glorious autumn day in the Midwest. As I drive along, I gulp down my 16.9 ounce bottle of water in less than five minutes. It has occurred to me that if the drivers behind me or next to me paid any attention, they would definitely have to wonder, why is this guy drinking so much, so quickly, at 8:45 in the morning? Let them think as they may, I have only one thing on my mind, and that is the sign that says, "STOP – your treatment requires a full bladder!"

After today's session, I asked Donna whether she knew what materials were used to make the mold which positions the legs during treatment? She told me that she did not know exactly what the material was, but that she would gladly show me, if I was interested, how the mold was made. Of course I was interested. I followed Donna into the CT room and she took a green piece of what looked like styrofoam and put it on the table. Its dimensions were about two feet by two feet square. It was approximately two inches thick and was firm to the touch. She attached a hose to it and air was blown into it. Now it became something resembling a pillow. It was now also quite soft. I placed my forearms into it and pushed down gently. Donna now let the air out and the mold shrunk down and closed around my forearms. In a real leg mold making session, the therapists help shape the material closely around the legs. Now the substance was quite hard and presented a perfect fit for my arms. She explained that by simply inflating and deflating this material, it could be used over and over again. This method made sense – efficient and economical, indeed.

I had to meet again with Dr. Sinclair today. I knew what to do. Just outside his office is a scale. I saw Tina, the medical assistant, standing and waiting for me by it. After emptying out my pockets and taking off my shoes, I stood absolutely still waiting for the verdict. "One pound up from last week," she declared. I was not pleased. My goal was to lose nine pounds in nine weeks. Obviously, I was not anywhere close to reaching my target.

Dr. Sinclair was his usual smiling self. "So, how's it going?" was his cheerful greeting. I had to tell him that for the last few days, it had not been going so well. The urge to pee came more and more frequently, but it was extremely difficult to get anything going, and then, drop-by-drop. In addition, there was a stinging, burning sensation even with the slightest trickle. I would possibly sit for nearly ten minutes on the toilet, and when I was finished with my meager expulsion, I felt absolutely exhausted.

"Knucklehead," Dr. Sinclair said to me with a smile on his face. "Why didn't you come to me sooner? You don't have to wait for the next scheduled meeting. I am here all the time. Just let me know that you want to see me. OK?" I nodded. "So," he continued, "taking three ibuprofens twice a day obviously didn't do it for you. I will prescribe something more potent for that. This medicine just loosens everything up down there. Now, how are you coming along with your stomach problems?"

"That has fortunately subsided," I told him. "I don't drink any coffee, tea, soda or juice, and I watch my spices. So far, so good."

Dr. Sinclair smiled again and said, "Good, let's go out and I will tell Tina to give you the prescription."

Once we were in the office he told her, "Please give Mr. Stefan the Tamsulosin prescription." We shook hands and he went back into his office. This medication must be prescribed very frequently, because Tina opened a drawer and pulled out a sheet on which she simply wrote my name in the space provided. The rest was already filled in – Tamsulosin HCL 0.4 mg capsule. Dr. Sinclair's signature was affixed at the bottom.

Wow, thirty-two treatments down, thirteen more to go. This is cause for celebration, and how do I celebrate? – by telling another one of my jokes.

A man sits down on a park bench. After a while, he notices that the man sitting at the other end of the bench seems very sad, very depressed. He speaks to the man asks, "My friend, you seem so very sad. Is something troubling you?"
The man answers softly, "My third wife just died."
"Your third wife just died? What happened to the first one?"
"She died eating poison mushrooms."
"And your second wife? What happened to her?"
"She also died eating poison mushroom."
"So, what happened to your third wife?"
"She fell down the stairs and broke her neck."
"Oh my, how did that happen?"
Slight pause.
"She didn't want to eat the mushrooms."

Day 33

Dressing room 3. Therapists: Donna and Brenda

During my years as a high school German teacher, I took my students on several trips to Germany, and our school also participated in a student exchange program with a school in Hamburg. When we went on our trips, my wife, parents and even other teachers often accompanied us. After my retirement, I was asked whether I couldn't arrange another trip for family and friends. This trip turned out to be the first of fifteen such trips that were to follow. I would make up an itinerary – cities, towns and landmarks – that I thought would be of interest to Americans. I would then contact our agent, who had made the arrangements for our previous school trips, and he would calculate the cost involved. This cost for twenty-five participants (a manageable number of people for us to handle) would include the flight, hotel, bus transportation and sightseeing. He would then make up a brochure describing the places we would visit, the names of the hotels where we would stay and the airline company. Everything was based on double occupancy, with a slightly higher cost for a single supplement. I would then share this information with the people who had shown an interest in going with us. I did the planning and my wife did all of the administrative work. I always said that we have such a happy marriage because we have the perfect division of labor: I do the talking; she does the labor.

Since we both speak German, our trips mostly concentrated on the German speaking countries. We did, however, cross the border often and visited placed like

Paris, Reims, Strasbourg and the Loire Valley. We crossed the Alps and saw Milan, Venice and Verona. One of our trips started in Brussels, that beautiful city in Belgium. We had lunch several times in Luxembourg City, Luxembourg and in Vaduz, Liechtenstein.

The reason I mention this is because I have made a game, a mental exercise, if you will, of recalling the places that we have been to – one trip at a time with all of the various stops in the proper order. So, when I can't sleep, or while here on the table, I pick a trip and relive it to the best of my ability. Since I am the one who makes up the itinerary, I usually have no problem getting the towns in order, but I can also name the hotels in each city that we stayed, and in my mind I can see the buildings and even the rooms in which we stayed.

While on the table in the vault today, I let this year's trip of a few months ago, run past me. There were twenty-eight of us and I could easily name each participant. I remember clearly that it was a bright Monday morning, 7:20 a.m., when the Lufthansa jet landed in Frankfurt, Germany. Our bus was waiting outside the terminal. I introduced the driver (whose name had been given to me prior to departure) and told our group that for the next ten days, this man would be the most important person on our trip. I also told everyone that José was not a bus driver, but a chauffeur. This differentiation is very important to these men. These chauffeurs know their way around all of the European countries. They speak four or five languages; they know all the highway rest stops; they know the best places to eat, where to go and where not to go. I have learned right from our first trip on that it was always wise to listen to what these experienced travelers had to say.

Since our last trip (two years ago) had gone more south and east from central Germany, I had planned a more westerly itinerary for this trip, because thirteen of this year's participants had also been on the last trip.

Our first stop was Rüdesheim on the Rhine River – a quaint city nestled among the vineyards of this famous wine-growing region. Our hotel was fifty yards from the river and from its terrace you had a beautiful view of the river and all of the tour boats and barges that moved back and forth on this busy river highway. If you took the cable car, which starts about two blocks up the hill, you could comfortably get to the highest point of the mountain. Here you could visit the famous Niederwald Denkmal – a huge statue of Germania, looking across the Rhine, telling the French not to cross into this territory. This monument was erected after the Franco-Prussian War in 1871.

We drove to the Loreley Cliff the next morning, where legend has it that a beautiful maiden jumped into the churning Rhine waters because her knight in shining armor had not returned from the war. And now she sits up there, sings her enchanting songs, and lures the sailors to their death.

We saw the famous corner in Koblenz where the Mosel River flows into the Rhine River. This is called Zum Deutschen Eck. We had lunch in Luxembourg once again and spent the night in Trier, the oldest city in Germany, founded by the Romans around the time of Christ. It was these Romans who built the impressive Porta Nigra (black gate), which still stands today as a reminder of their glorious past.

We stopped in Baden-Baden, the famous spa town, and playground of kings, queens and artists. The casino is world famous, and this is where Dostoyevsky wrote his fascinating story, *The Gambler*.

On to Freiburg, in the heart of the Black Forest. The cathedral was started in the fourteenth century, and since there is always scaffolding around this magnificent structure, you could easily believe that the building has never been finished.

A quick stop was made after breakfast the next morning at the beautiful lake, Titisee, named after Emperor Titus. This town, Titsee-Neustadt, is famous for its Schwarzwälder Kirsch Torte (Black Forest Cherry Cake), and so we all indulged in a slice of cake and a second cup of coffee. This area is also famous for its Cherry Brandy, which gives the cake a most unique and delicious taste.

The next two days were spent in Lucerne, Switzerland. We took a relaxing two-hour boat ride on Lake Lucerne to a town at the far end of it, where we boarded the world's steepest cog rail, which took us up to the top of Mt. Pilatus. It was cloudy and brisk up there, but once in a while you could see the blue lake and the city of Lucerne far below.

On our way to Lindau, a beautiful city on Lake Constance, we stopped in Vaduz, Liechtenstein, one of the smallest, but most interesting cities and countries in the world, famous for its collection of postage stamps.

We saw the Wieskirche, the most splendid Rococo church in southern Germany. We visited the picturesque town of Oberammergau, with its colorfully painted house facades; the town is famous for its world-renowned Passion plays that are performed every ten years.

Finally, we stayed in Bad Tölz for three days, a quaint village in the Bavarian Alps. From here we took excursions to Passau and Herrenchiemsee. In Passau, we took a boat ride on the Danube River aboard the sparkling Swarovski Kristallschiff. The entire ship is decorated with Swarovski crystals – a truly unique experience. On our final day we visited the Herrenchiemsee Castle, built on an island by Ludwig II of Bavaria. It is an imitation of the Versailles Palace in France, except that mad King Ludwig had to make the famous Hall of Mirrors a little larger than the original one.

After ten exciting, but still relaxing days, Lufthansa flew us home from Munich.

I can recall most of our trips perfectly, and in my mind, I can see all of those wonderful places again and again.

The world is beautiful, and I am happy that I can recollect all of the marvelous places that we have been to at any time I want.

So, my dear linear accelerator, wipe out and kill everything that is eating away at me, scorch that walnut-sized gland down there – but my memories, my beautiful memories of wonderful places, of good times with dear friends, that is something that you or anybody or anything else will never be able to take from me.

Day 34

Dressing room 3. Therapists: Donna and Brenda

The side effects of the radiation therapy have now become very real – not only at certain times and during specific activities – now there is a constant reminder that there is something wrong inside of me and that something is being done about it. There is now a constant tingle in the prostate region, and this tingling extends, at times, right into the (p word). It is not painful, but it does remind me that I am a patient, and that for my own good something is being destroyed inside of me.

Although the doctor had discussed the possible side effects of this treatment (I say "possible" because not all men react in the same way), I decided to consult the internet. Here is what I found:

Side Effects of External Radiation Therapy

Intestinal Side Effects:

During and after radiation treatment for prostate cancer, there may be diarrhea and/or rectal pain, irritable bowels, sometimes, bloody stools.

Urinary Side Effects:

Burning pain while urinating, occasional blood in the urine and an increased frequency in the urge to urinate are seen in patients who have radiation treatment for prostate cancer.

Other Side Effects:

The ACR mentions dermatological side effects like dryness of the skin, with or without temporary or permanent hair loss, over the areas targeted by the radiation therapy. Other side effects listed by the ACR are fatigue and lymphedema, or fluid buildup in the legs and genitals.

Impotence:

Impotence shows a delayed onset after radiation therapy, according to the ACR, quite the contrary to surgery, where impotence is immediate and may actually improve over time.

So, where am I at after thirty-four treatments?

Category 1 – I experienced the onset of diarrhea, but a daily dose of Metamucil has eliminated this problem.

Category 2 – Increase in the urge to urinate has definitely occurred and there is some pain associated with it.

Category 3 – I have, up to this point, not noticed any of these symptoms.

Category 4 – I respectfully request to be allowed to withhold indefinitely any comment on this issue.

I do, however, not want to end this very important aspect on this note. So, here is a related joke, also from the internet.

> *"Doctor," the embarrassed man said, "I have a sexual problem. I can't get it up for my wife anymore."*
> *"Mr. Brown," replies the doctor, "bring her back with you tomorrow and let me see what I can do."*
> *The next day the worried fellow returns with his wife.*
> *"Take off your clothes, Mrs. Brown," the doctor instructs her. "Now turn all the way around. Lie down, please. Uh-huh. I see. You may put your clothes back on."*
> *The doctor takes the husband aside. "You're perfectly healthy," he states. "Your wife didn't give me an erection either."*

After I read this joke again, I thought that it would be wise of me to write an apology to all the women who might wind up reading my story. But the more I thought about it, the more I became inclined not to do that. And I will tell you why: The women that I know, every one of them, are beautiful, each in her own unique way. These women are intelligent, self-confident and multi-talented. They are not the shy, mousy and subservient females of yesterday. They know where they stand and are not shy to express it. They have proven that they can do any job a man can do – they are doctors, company executives, drive buses, and can fly into outer space, etc. etc.

I belong to a book group where the attendance at the once a month meeting usually consists of fourteen to fifteen women and two men, me being one of them. I enjoy these meetings, because we read books that lend themselves to great discussions, and because these women have wonderful insights and can speak from experiences of which the average man has not even the slightest inkling.

I'll come right out and say it: I enjoy the company of women, all those lively, witty and charming women. I am sure that I am not the first man to recognize the civilizing effect that the contact with women has on us, sometimes, brutish creatures.

I, for one, am grateful for all of the wonderful women in my life, and I thank each one for bringing that little extra touch of delight into my life every day.

Day 35

Dressing room 3. Therapists: Ted and Brenda

It rained today as I set out for the clinic. No, it did not just rain – it poured. As I gulped down my water while driving, the windshield wipers could barely keep up with the amount of water that was being dumped on them.

Water is a necessity of life here on earth. Our bodies are made up of more than 70% of it. More than half of the earth's surface is covered with it. We drink it, we cook with it, we wash our clothes with it, we shower and bathe with it; we simply need it for everything.

I have always loved water. There was a little pond not far from our house, and a quiet brook that gently flowed through the meadows. We swam in it in the summer and skated on the pond in the winter. In my younger days, I loved nothing more than spending a day at the beach.

But that was then and this is now. Water, more specifically, running, gushing water, has become my daily tormentor. Let me explain why: Many years ago, I had to go for a blood test. When my name was called, a nurse handed me a plastic cup and told me that she needed a urine specimen. I told her that this might take a while since I didn't know that a urine sample would be required and that I had emptied my bladder just a few minutes ago. She told me that I should go into the bathroom and let the water run into the sink. This would stimulate me to be able to urinate. I did as I was told, but I thought this was a dumb idea, some kind of old wives' tale. I have washed my car hundreds of times using a hose that gushed out water in a powerful stream. I have taken who knows how many showers under splashing jets of water. I have stood on the side of the Schaffhausen waterfall, the largest waterfall in Europe. I have stood so close to the pounding waters of Niagara Falls that I could feel my feet vibrate from the power of that mighty torrent of water. I have watched the water gush forth beneath me as I stood atop Hoover Dam. If all that powerful, gushing, pounding water did not make me pee, how could this gentle, controlled flow of water accomplish this act? And it didn't! After some serious concentration, I was finally able to barely do what was required of me.

But as I said before, that was then and this is now. I get up in the morning, turn on the water to brush my teeth, and I turn it off again because I gotta go. I let the hot water run so I can shave, I turn it off again because I gotta go. I make sure that my bladder is empty before I take a shower, because recently it happened that I barely made it back to the toilet before the shower floor would have been sprinkled by something other than cleansing water. Not long ago, my wife wanted to replant one of our potted plants into the garden. I dug the hole, she carefully put the flower in the right position; we added the dirt and tapped it down. She then said, "Make sure to give it a good soaking so the roots will take hold." Well, I pulled out the garden hose, let the water run, found the right setting and began to water the newly planted flower. I didn't get far. The gushing water and the feel of it running through the hose put a quick end to my initial watering attempt. I ran into the house and came back a few minutes later to finish the job.

A far more serious and nearly very unpleasant experience occurred a few days ago. I had gone grocery shopping, and as I came out of the store, I felt the first urge to go. But no, being the macho man, I decided that I might as well get some gas for the car so that I would not have to go out later to fill the tank. I prepaid my twenty dollars inside the station, went out to my pump and inserted the nozzle into the gas tank opening. I then proceeded to tank up my car. When the nozzle pumped out that hard flowing stream of gasoline, something just went crazy inside of me. By the time the meter indicated that three dollars worth of gas had been pumped, I felt that I had to go bad. By the time it reached eight dollars, I knew I was in big trouble. At twelve dollars, I began to cross my legs, first one way and then another. What should I do? I did not just want to shut off the hose and run inside the gas station with the hose still stuck in the gas tank. That did not seem a wise thing to do. So, I pushed down as hard as I could on the lever, but the numbers on the pump didn't move any faster. It seemed like an eternity before the dial showed nineteen twenty-five, nineteen-fifty, nineteen seventy-five. As soon as the numbers stopped at twenty dollars, I ripped out the hose, slammed it back into the pump, gave the gas cap one turn and ran into the gas station, hoping and praying that the one washroom inside was not occupied. It wasn't and I made it without an embarrassing accident.

Is there a lesson to be learned from all of this? The lesson I learned is that when you are young and healthy, be patient with the elderly, be understanding of their ailments, be helpful whenever you can. Now, I don't want to preach, but someday you may be the one (as I am now) who will need all the love and kindness that you can possibly get.

Day 36

Dressing room 2. Therapists: Ted and Brenda

I was just ready to enter the building when the man who receives his treatment ahead of me stepped out and said, "Hi." I asked him where he was in his treatment and he told me that he had five more sessions to go. I told him that I was right behind him with ten more to follow. I asked him how the treatment was affecting him. He shrugged his shoulders and said that everything was all right. The only thing that was different was that he got up several times during the night to pee. I told him that I had the same problem, but that at times there was a considerable burning pain associated with it. He nodded and said with a wink, "When that happens to me, I know who to blame. I love to have my hamburger smothered with onions, and I will have my ribs in a spicy barbecue sauce. And I will not do without my chocolate. I eat chocolate every day." I told him that I tried to watch my intake, but that at times, this was definitely a real challenge. You see I love coffee. I used to make two lattés a day for my wife and myself. After months of experimenting with different coffees, I have come to the conclusion that the Lavazza brand espresso (black can) gives us the most satisfying coffee experience, with the exception perhaps, of sitting in a Viennese café, sipping one of the many coffee creations for which this magnificent city is rightfully famous. "Well, what'cha gonna do?" he asked rhetorically, "You gotta keep on living, don't you?"

I couldn't agree more with him!

After that pleasant beginning to my day, I think it is appropriate for me to tell my fourth and final joke.

Two friends, who had not seen each other for a long time, finally meet and they talk about the past. After a while, one man notices that his friend seemed rather morose and downtrodden. After observing this for a while, he finally asks him if there is anything wrong. His friend replies, "Well, I'm broke, absolutely bankrupt." His friend is amazed and asks, "How did this happen? I heard that you had become a rich man, actually a very wealthy man."
"That's true," his friend replied.
"So what happened?" his friend asked again.
The man responded, "I spent most of my money on booze and broads – the rest I just wasted."

Day 37

Dressing room 3. Therapists: Ted and Brenda

When I told the therapists that I was going to keep a journal of my daily experiences here at the clinic, and that the resulting story, along with a few others that I have written, might possibly get published (I have already published two other books), they were very enthusiastic about this project and volunteered to help me in every way that they could. Pat told me that she had always wanted to write, and that she had a subject in mind (it was work-related and her chosen title sounded intriguing). I told her to go ahead and do it and not to worry about how it may turn out. "Give it a try," I said, "you may just be surprised by what you get." She smiled, but stayed non-committal. I hope she does it.

I have always felt that doing something, no matter how amateurishly is better than just being an observer on the sideline. Be active, do something. It really doesn't matter how good you are at it. If you like to paint, then do it, even though you know very well that you will never be another Renoir or Picasso. If you like to sing, join a choir – your singing most likely deserves to be heard by others. And if you like to write, then write. You may never be a Hemingway or Tolstoy. The fact that you will probably never write the great American novel should not stop you from doing that where your passion lies.

The beginning is always the hardest, and you may be disappointed at what you produce at first. Take a non-credit course at your local junior college; check whether your library doesn't have a writers group. You are not alone in your desire to do something creative.

My greatest reward came through my involvement in music. While in high school, I learned the rudiments of first position violin playing. I played in the school orchestra, but I never became very good. Later, I met a man in our church who was a very good amateur violinist. We began to play duets together, and later our church organist joined us and accompanied us on the piano. Soon a young man who was a fairly decent cellist rounded out our quartet. The problem was that we could not find much music that was written for two violins, cello and piano. It was at this time that I began to arrange the cello part, mostly taken from the bass line of the piano, to fit into the music we were playing. After a while, I began to write my own pieces for our ensemble. Sure, they were simple, especially the piano part, but I felt that every new piece I composed was better than the last one.

When I arrived at the high school where I spent the last eighteen years of my teaching career, I noticed that the school did not have an orchestra (it had the usual bands and choruses), but no ensemble with strings. Then one day I saw a student walking down the hall with a violin case in his hand. I asked him whether he knew of other string players in this school. He told me that he knew of a girl who also played the violin and that there was a boy who played the cello.

I had an announcement made over the school's intercom system inviting anyone who played a string instrument to meet with me in my homeroom after school. Seven students showed up. We formed an ensemble and played in my room once a week after school. The following year, we had ten students – including a viola player and a bass player. We also had an outstanding pianist. Soon we had twelve musicians, then fifteen, and after seven years of this after school music making, our number had grown to eighteen. Some of these young musicians were quite accomplished on their instruments. Our "String Ensemble" was invited to play at assemblies, faculty dinners and we even received an invitation to play at city hall. People were always surprised that these musicians playing Mozart, Bach, Pachelbel and arrangements of modern pieces, were Chicago public school students and not youngsters from some elite suburban school.

After I had pleaded for many years to make "strings" part of the student course offering, the orchestra finally became officially part of the curriculum.

Since I am the founder of the orchestra program at this school, one string player is annually awarded a scholarship in my name. I have been invited to conduct and perform one of my own compositions with the orchestra at their spring and fall concerts.

This initial, so very amateurish beginning has now benefited hundreds of students at this school. There are currently more than 250 students enrolled in the string program and the Advanced Orchestra is considered to be one of the best in the entire state.

When I started this ensemble, I had no idea that some day it would be so successful. It just goes to show, as I have always believed, that anything done with love and from the heart will always succeed beyond your wildest dreams.

Day 38

Dressing room 1. Therapists: Ted and Brenda

One thing I like about this clinic is that all the people I meet, right from the friendly greeting in the morning from the three ladies in the office, to seeing the three therapists and the chief therapist outside the vault, to the friendly wave from the nutritionist as I walk past her office; everyone is cheerful and upbeat. I can tell that this is not an act put on for us by the patients. Their smiles and their friendly demeanor are genuine, and this leads me to the following conclusion: these people like their jobs. They enjoy what they are doing.

As Donna and I came out of the vault today, there was no one in the waiting area. I took advantage of this situation and asked her right out whether she liked her job, whether it was meeting all of the expectations that she must have had while preparing for this demanding profession.

"Oh, yes," she answered, "I like my job very much. I like the people I work with, and I like what I do. You meet so many interesting people. Most of all, however, the feeling that you get from doing this job is that you have done something useful."

Something useful – I liked that. What these people do down here is way beyond useful – it is life saving.

Except for the part-time jobs that I've had during my high school and college years, I can honestly say that I was one of those lucky people who really enjoyed his work –

looked forward to going there every day. Teaching is indeed a noble profession, and I was very fortunate to spend the last eighteen years of my teaching career in a school where I was actually able to teach and not just try to control the kids for fifty minutes at a time. I taught in the renowned International Baccalaureate Program. This program uses a curriculum that has been developed by a group of international educators. The point is that the children of parents who move a lot (consulates, ambassadors, business executives, etc.) are taught a curriculum that meets the highest international standards. However, the program is also open to local students who are able to meet the demanding entrance requirements.

I loved being with these kids aged thirteen through nineteen, and I taught students from all over the world. This made every day interesting. One could never know what to expect on any given day. I also liked the fact that since I was the only German teacher in the school, the students spent all four years of their foreign language study with me. I knew them and they knew me. It was a pleasure to watch a kid of thirteen or fourteen blossom into a mature young man or woman. Often the changes were very surprising, not only in physical appearance, but also in maturity. I remember that one of the silliest and downright goofy (but smart) kids in my class became a rabbi. I heard that another one of my students, a shy and quiet boy, worked his way through college as a male stripper.

It is not surprising for me to turn on my computer in the morning and find an email from one of my former students. At the moment, one of them is working at the embassy in Prague; another works for the American consulate in Vienna. Another former student, a shy and quiet boy from India, has contacted me recently and asked if we could meet for coffee. We met and he told me that he had become a cardio-vascular surgeon, and that he was leaving soon to spend a year in a hospital on the outskirts of Frankfurt, Germany. Here he was going to learn how to do a new bypass procedure, which had been developed at this hospital, and then teach this new technique to doctors back here in the states. He had taken more German classes in college and we conducted our entire conversation in German. You cannot imagine how proud I was to see my work play at least a small role in making this man into what he has become today.

Most of all, however, I enjoyed being with those young people because we had so much fun together and anything could happen at almost any time.

One day, a student sneezed in class and I said, "Gesundheit." Another student raised his hand and said, "Herr Stefan, how would you say that in German?" The whole class howled.

Every person is happy when he or she feels that his or her work is appreciated. On the day I retired, I believe I was paid the biggest compliment that any teacher could ever receive. One of my senior students gave me a big hug and said, "You are the only teacher I know that nobody hates." I loved it, because that is something that not many teachers can say about themselves.

Day 39

Dressing room 2. Therapists: Ted and Donna

There is a saying that states, "Beauty is in the eye of the beholder." That is most certainly true, but in my opinion, the statement doesn't go far enough. I would say, "Everything is in the eye of the beholder." I think that it is fair to say that what we see in our life is perceived from the perspective of our upbringing, level of education, economic situation; from our religious, racial and ethnic background. Everything we see is tinged in some way by who we are and by how we see ourselves in this world.

This thought came to me as once again I entered dressing room 2. I had noticed it before, briefly wondered about it, but never given it any real thought. This is what I am talking about: Each of the four dressing rooms, and one of the two bathrooms, has black and white photographs of various international cityscapes hung on the walls. I don't know who decorated these tiny rooms in this way, or whether that person had considered or was even aware, of what these rooms were to be used for.

In one room hangs a picture of Paris with the Eiffel Tower protruding elegantly, but firmly, into a cloudy sky. On another wall is a picture of the dome of Sacre Coeur, with its gently curved round tip.

Another room features the British Parliament Building, with its massive, strong Big Ben tower dominating everything around it.

There are two pictures in another room. One is of the Twin Towers of the New York World Trade Center; the other, the Empire State Building, rising ever upward, tall and proud. But my favorite is the lighthouse tower in the last room; round, strong and confident. Its mushroom-shaped top just makes it look like – well, I'll leave that up to your imagination.

Okay – maybe it's just me. Maybe the 38 radiation treatments that I have received so far have something to do with it, but that's the way it is. This is what I see on those walls – given my current condition. And are these strong, upright, firm and erect structures really what tired old men, who are bombarded daily with shriveling and shrinkage causing destructive rays, need to see at this stage in their lives?

I wonder if these pictures have intrigued any of the other men. Maybe not, but that just goes to show that we all see the world around us differently.

The following joke demonstrates my point perfectly. I think that I might have heard it in one of the psychology classes that I took while in college.

A psychiatrist is giving the Rorschach (inkblot) test to a patient. The doctor holds up the first picture and asks, "What do you see in this picture?"
Patient: "I see two people having sex."
Doctor: "OK, and what do you see in this picture?"
Patient: "I see two people having sex."
Doctor: "Uh-huh, and what do you see in this picture?"
Patient: "I see two people having sex."

This goes on for some time. Always the same question and always the same answer.

Finally, the doctor can't take it anymore and he yells at the patient, "What's wrong with you? Do you always have to see two people having sex?"

And the patient yells back even more indignantly, "What's wrong with ME? YOU'RE the one showing me the dirty pictures!!!"

Day 40

Dressing room 3. Therapists: Donna and Brenda

If you enter the clinic from the left of the building, you have to walk all the way through the waiting room that serves the urology offices on the first floor to get to the elevator on the other side. This is where my wife and I had sat two times; first, to consult with Dr. Delgado, my urologist, and secondly, to have the biopsy performed.

If you enter by the door on the right side of the building, you still come into this waiting room, but the elevator is immediately to your right. Every morning, the number of people who are already here waiting to see the urologist amazes me. But it is not only the number of people I see sitting here when I enter, or when I leave, (and there are always new people), I am also amazed at the condition of some of these people. To be sure, there are always some men there who are younger than I am and who seem to be in pretty good physical shape. But there are men who have walked in steadying themselves on their walking canes. Others sit there with their walkers in front of them, and some are even there in wheel chairs. I feel sorry for these men, because of whatever else ails them, and I am sure that they have multiple other physical problems; do they have to be plagued by yet another ailment, whatever it is that brings them here?

And it is not only the men that I feel sorry for. I see them arriving in cars driven by their wives. They help them into the building; they hand them a napkin for their runny noses, and they go with their husband when his name is called. Some of these men would not make it on their own. And do these women not have enough problems of their own already? Some of them seem to be suffering themselves. So, besides all of the work that has already fallen on them due to their husbands' age and condition, do they still need this on top of all of the problems they already face?

And once these men get to see the doctor, what will they get to hear? That their ailment is not so serious and can be treated? That their ailment will require major surgery? That there may be some help, but that there is really nothing much that can still be done?

The elevator that goes only down from here is a slow elevator, and that gives me ample time to look at this scene. It is a sad and depressing sight. Hardly anyone pays attention to the two television monitors which both broadcast the same program. Sometimes I press the elevator button again, although I know fully well that this will not make it arrive any faster.

Many years ago, I heard this phrase quite often, "Life's a bitch and then you die." I never liked this phrase, although I was aware that usually it was merely said about some minor mishap a person may have experienced. But it still bothered me every time I heard it. Part of that statement is definitely true, the part, "and then you die." It is the first part, "life's a bitch," with which I simply cannot agree.

No, life is not a bitch. Life is a sacred gift that has been bestowed on us, the living. Life is meant to be lived to the fullest, and every minute of it is to be treasured. I know that some people will now object and say, yes, that is easy to say when you are young and healthy; when you are well off and don't have to worry about next month's rent or how to pay the next gas bill. Isn't it interesting, that most of the "bitching" comes from people who have nothing to bitch about? They are annoyed by minor inconveniences that, seen from a broader perspective, are absolutely meaningless. I have seen real poverty first hand, but I have also seen people like my parents, who faced their hardships bravely, who had the courage and faith to start a new life in a strange and distant land. They worked hard and were grateful for every improvement in their life. We see this repeated thousands of times every day, not only here, but also all over the world. It is these people who treasure life the most, who rejoice at every accomplishment they or their children, may achieve. They celebrate the good moments in life, no matter how infrequently these moments may occur.

There is another saying that touched me very deeply the first time I heard it. "I felt sorry for myself because I had no shoes, until I saw a man who had no feet." I do have shoes, very soft and cushioned walking shoes. These shoes take me comfortably to wherever I want to go. But I have been given another, even more comfortable pair of shoes, the shoes that take me on my course through life – and for this, I am eternally grateful!

Day 41

Dressing room 3. Therapists: Ted and Donna

Everything about the weekend was beautiful: the weather, the food, the ride to the forest preserve where the trees are at their colorful best – everywhere orange, brown, gold and red. Mother Nature was signaling the change of seasons in a magnificent display of radiant colors.

Everything out there was fantastic, but inside of me – well, it wasn't that great. No, it wasn't great at all. As a matter of fact, I was miserable. This weekend had been the roughest time since the treatment began. The trouble, of course, was the "flow." Here again is a perfect example of how we take things for granted as long as everything works well. I don't remember how many times I got up during the night, but it wasn't just the inconvenience of having my sleep constantly interrupted (actually I didn't sleep at all in the early morning hours), but there was pain, real pain, which made me break out in a sweat as I tried to squeeze and push whatever I could out of my bladder.

Since Dr. Sinclair had called me a "knucklehead" for waiting to see him until the appointed time, I decided to see him as soon as possible. He had told me that he would not be in the office this Tuesday (my appointed day). As soon as I arrived at the office on Monday morning, I told Jan, the nurse that I would like to see the doctor after my treatment. She told me that Dr. Sinclair had already left, but that Dr. Petrarch was taking his place and that she would see me.

Dr. Petrarch turned out to be a delightful lady, probably just a few years younger than me. She was elegantly dressed and had an absolutely stunning diamond ring on her right hand. Her greatest feature, however, may just have been her smooth and lovely skin. She made an immediate, most positive impression.

She inquired how things have been going, and I told her my current situation. After she had listened to my complaints, she spoke with a gentle voice and with a charming accent that I could not place.

She had a folder in front of her and occasionally glancing into it, she said, "I see that you started with one Tamsulosin a day—that's the FLOMAX. Then you took that with three ibuprofens. After that you took the ibuprofen twice a day, and now you are at FLOMAX twice a day and the ibuprofen once. Is that right?

I nodded, "That's correct." She continued, "After all of this, it might be a good idea to try something else. There is a stronger medicine available that's called RAPAFLO. I think you should give that a try. Where is your urologist?" I told her that he was just a floor above us, right here in this building. "That's great," she replied, "I will ask the nurse to get you some samples. They always have them. There is no reason for you to buy them."

So this is where it stands. Tonight, a half hour after dinner, I will take the RAPAFLO and wait and see what will happen.

I took the FLOMAX - and nothing flowed to the max. Now I will take the RAPAFLO, but I'm not holding my breath for the rapid flow to happen.

You got to leave it to the marketing people at the pharmaceutical companies. The names of the products are very descriptive and let you have high expectations.

94

I try to be an optimist about everything in life. I know that the "flow" will eventually return, but feeling the way I do, I wish that this would happen as soon as possible – tomorrow would be real good!

Day 42

Dressing room 4. Therapists: Donna and Brenda

Dr. Sinclair is back and I went to see him right away, even before my treatment. I explained my situation and he asked me if there was a burning sensation during my efforts to pee. I told him that there was. I also told him that during the last few days my blood pressure had gone straight through the roof: 201/97 and 195/95 and 179/90. Dr. Sinclair told me that after my treatment, I should come back and provide a urine sample, just to make sure I didn't have a bladder infection. And that is what I did.

Some time ago, I asked whether I had met all the people who worked here in the Center for Prostate Cancer. I was told no, that on Mondays, Wednesdays and Fridays there was another lady here – Roseanne, the office manager. I asked Tina whether she could find out if I could see this Roseanne and introduce myself to her. She came back in a few seconds and told me that I should go right into her office, which is on the right, almost hidden from view.

When I entered, I was glad to see that Pat was there, too. Roseanne rose from her chair, shook my hand, and before I could say anything, she said, "So, you are writing a book about your experiences here." That took me by surprise, because I had not anticipated that anyone had told her about my daily journal. "No," I replied, "I'm not really writing a book about it, but if I add the five short stories that I have already written, that could perhaps produce a thin book. Of course, everything will depend on the publisher. If he likes the material, then maybe this will appear in print." And then I had to tell how I came up with this idea and how I was going about it. I also mentioned that Pat had already agreed to look over the manuscript to see if I got the technical aspects correct. Then Pat told me that Roseanne was quite an accomplished editor. That was great news, and I asked her immediately if she wouldn't mind looking over the manuscript too once it was finished. She agreed to do it. I was overjoyed to now have the help of two such experienced people at my disposal.

As I left the office, Tina told me that I did not have a bladder infection and that Dr. Sinclair wanted me to take two FLOMAX tablets in the evening, and also that I should see my own doctor about the high blood pressure.

As soon as I got home, I called Dr. Bauer on his pager at the hospital. He called back and I told him about my blood pressure situation. He told me that he would call his office to put me down as his last patient for the day.

I saw Dr. Bauer that evening. The blood pressure reading on my right arm was 130/80, and the reading using my left arm was 130/70. Now this was strange and both of us could not come up with an answer for the discrepancy. I assured Dr. Bauer that, after 42 visits to the clinic, I certainly was not nervous or tense about receiving the radiation treatment. Dr. Bauer asked me to continue to monitor this problem and let him know if there were any changes.

Day 43

Dressing room 4. Therapists: Ted and Donna

As soon as I took my ID card and the attached dressing room key from the counter, I realized that today was going to be a very special day. There, in the office, I saw Megan, Jan and Tina going about their work, but they were all dressed in dark blue police uniforms. Jan asked me to come into their office. She pointed to the floor and told me to walk a straight line. The problem with that was that they had drawn a line that curved sharply to the left and to the right. I told them that I loved their uniforms, and they all came forward and had me read what it said on the patches that were sewn on the left breast of their shirts. Megan's patch read, "Captain Morgan," Jan's read, "Miranda Wright," and Tina's read, "Eva Dense." They all looked great in their uniforms. However, that was not the end of it. They brought Dr. Sinclair out of his office to show me his outfit. He also wore a policeman's uniform, but on his breast patch it read, "Oliver Klozhoff." I had to think about that for a second or two, but then it became very clear – all of her clothes off. It's good to see a doctor with a sense of humor. I was then taken to Roseanne's office where I also met Pat. Roseanne got up immediately and said, "Can you guess?" She was wearing a Chicago Bears jersey and she picked up a portable fan. That wasn't too difficult. Pat proved to be a little harder to figure out. She wore jeans and a brown and yellow colored top. I finally got it – she was a cougar. I am sure you all know that the word cougar, besides referring to the animal, also means an older woman who goes after younger men. Pat looked wonderful in her outfit, but she is much too young to be that kind of cougar.

When I went back to the treatment area, I noticed that Brenda and Donna both wore the same outfits – the Ghost Buster uniforms, except that it said "Cancer Buster" on their ghost buster suits. The star of the show, however, was Ted. He emerged from the vault wearing a big, round and green bubble around his chest and midsection, and on it was written, "Tumor." His face was smeared with black and green markings making it very clear that tumors and cancer are very ugly things.

A table had been set up in the treatment area waiting room – it was loaded with cheese, cold cuts, cakes, cookies and donuts. Freshly brewed coffee and soft drinks were also available. It was interesting to see that former patients had returned to say "Hi" to the people who had treated them in the past – what a powerful testament to the beautiful relationship that had developed between the patients and the people who cared for them.

I consider myself very fortunate that I was directed to this place to be cured of the disease that is within me. Yes, it is a highly sophisticated, technologically and scientifically most advanced machine that does much of the work, but without the caring involvement of dedicated and loving people, this therapy would by far not be as successful as it is for all of us.

Day 44

Dressing room 1. Therapists: Donna and Brenda

After today's treatment session, I asked Donna and Brenda whether tomorrow, on my last day, I would get a "diploma," like the one I saw a man carry out with him several days ago. Donna smiled and said mischievously, "Well, in your case we may just have to add a few extra treatments." I was not to be outdone and so I responded, "Okay, if I can choose the treatment, I will gladly come." And now Brenda added laughingly, "We'll have to see about that."

Now, under different circumstances, I would never have dared to say anything that suggestive to women whom I had known for only such a short time, but this was different. Donna and Brenda, as well as the rest of the staff, had time and time again shown that they had a wonderful sense of humor. Come to think of it, a great sense of humor had to be almost a prerequisite in order to be able to do this job. Hour after hour, day after day, these highly trained and skillful health care professionals have to deal with a never-ending stream of old, sick men. I am sure that not all of them are pleasant to deal with. Some may be bitter, uncooperative and resentful. And then again, some may try too hard to be funny and their humor may be obnoxious and offensive. Whatever the case may be, I have seen everyone down here to be as pleasant and upbeat as they could possibly be. I, for one, appreciate that very much.

Then it was time for my scheduled appointment with Dr. Sinclair. I had to wait for him for just a few minutes before he came out of the room where my Fiducial Marker Placement Procedure had been performed. He closed the door behind him, sat down opposite me and asked, "So, how's it going?" I told him that everything was all right, but that I thought that I had reached the "numb nut" stage. He gave me a questioning look. "For days now," I explained, "it feels down there, especially in bed at night, as if I had just been kicked in the old cojones."

Dr. Sinclair grinned, "You are now at the most intense stage of the "sunburn." That will gradually subside after your last treatment."

He then told me that tomorrow we would go over what needed to be done for my post-therapy follow-ups.

Day 45

Dressing room 4. Therapists: Donna and Brenda

Although I left the house at 8:45 as I always do, and even though I had my 16.9 oz. water bottle set in the cup holder of my car, there was something different about this morning's ride to the Center for Prostate Cancer. On the seat next to me lay a bouquet of red roses and standing on the floor in a gift pouch was a bottle of Kentucky Bourbon for Ted. The rose bouquet held eight roses, one for each of the wonderful ladies that I had met in the course of the last nine weeks.

Megan, Jan, Tina and Pat were in the office when I arrived and were pleasantly surprised by the flowers. They hugged and thanked me as I explained that one rose was meant for each of them. Megan went and got a vase and arranged the flowers most skillfully.

Unfortunately, Ted had not been able to come to work today, so I left the pouch with Donna, who assured me that he would get my present.

After this, my final treatment, Donna and Brenda helped me off the table, and presented me with my diploma. It is a nicely printed sheet with an elegantly designed border. On the top it reads, "YOU DID IT! Presented to Helmut Stefan. Congratulations for completing your radiation treatment." Beneath that, it lists all of the names of the people involved in carrying out the therapy.

I also received a sticker, like a magnet, that you could hang on your refrigerator. It is white and has the yellow and black radiation-warning symbol on it. Above it is written in red "I survived a ride on the..." and then in big blue letters beneath it, "Linear Accelerator."

Donna and Brenda hugged me and said they enjoyed working with me. I, in turn, thanked them for making all of this a pleasant experience.

Back in the main office, Tina and I decided on my next visit, in about a month, and she gave me a form for taking a blood test, specifically concentrating on the PSA level. I was also given a questionnaire, which I was to fill out before I would see Dr. Sinclair. It was a form that asked the patient to rate the various services from excellent to poor. Needless to say, I checked off excellent in each category. On the back page, I wrote that the entire staff should be commended for the outstanding work that was done here and for the personal attention that each patient receives.

My visit with Dr. Sinclair was brief. He asked me if everything was all right. I assured him that it was. He told me that as time progressed, I may want to cut back on the FLOMAX and go to one pill a day, but I should regulate that as I see necessary.

We shook hands and he told me that he would see me in a month.

My way out was accompanied by cheerful "goodbyes," "see you in a month," "take care of yourself," and "thank you."

As I waited for the elevator, I was very well aware that an important phase of my life had come to an end.

There certainly was reason to rejoice that the treatment had been successfully carried out and that soon I could expect some of these truly bothersome side effects to subside, and yet.... I felt a touch of melancholy as I waited for that slow contraption to take me back up and away from the people that I respect, admire and of whom I have become very fond.

Reflections from the Vault

My Therapists

All those people above,
They don't know what you do,
But we who come down here,
We appreciate you!

Plea

Oh, prostate, my prostate
Why can't you see?
All that I want
Is to take a good pee!

Metamorphosis

My friends, I have been shaven,
Oh what pleasure, oh what joy!
Up here I look like an old man,
Down there – like a little boy!

Burn, Baby, Burn!

I cannot see nor hear you,
You strong and radiant beam,
But when I'm on the potty,
At times I could just scream.

I know that you will heal me,
I know all will be well,
But when I try to tinkle,
I wish you'd go to hell.

So, go ahead and burn me,
I know I will survive,
And soon now I will leave here,
Rejoicing and alive.

Hindsight

I've been stuck from the front
And probed from the rear.
"Give it no thought,
You have nothing to fear."
I can say that now,
Now that it's done.
But while it is happ'ning,
It sure ain't much fun!

106

You are not alone

Pale man on the table
Looking straight ahead,
I wonder what you're thinking,
What goes through your head?

Old man on the table,
I wonder what you'd say,
If I gently asked you,
"My friend, do you pray?"

Sick man on the table,
Forget past woes and strife,
Always, please, remember –
Where there is hope, there is Life!

Facts and Figures

Number of external radiation treatments: 45

Amount of time spent on table: Approximately 7 hours

Attending Therapists:

Ted and Donna: 14 times

Ted and Brenda: 13 times

Donna and Brenda: 18 times

Dressing rooms used:

Dressing room 1: 8 times

Dressing room 2: 7 times

Dressing room 3: 18 times

Dressing room 4: 12 times

Number of miles driven round trip: 360 miles

Amount of water consumed before sessions: Approximately 6 gallons

Weight lost: 3 pounds

Nighttime visits to the bathroom: 2471 (just kidding, but sometimes it sure seemed like it).

Other Suggested Titles

My friends thought that "The Full Bladder Club" was a funny title for my little literary effort. I encouraged them to come up with other names that could apply to all of us men who are going through this experience. This is a partial list of their creative effort:

Tricky Tricklers

Drooping Ding-Dongs

Prostrate Prostates

Noodle Doodles

Trickle Pickles

Busting Bladders

Petered-out Peckers

Now, there were a few others, but I thought it wise not to list them here in fear of offending some of the more sensitive readers. If you would like to hear them, just ask. I will gladly share them with you, but only if you promise not to blush.

Sayings I jotted down during these nine weeks:

Those who love deeply never grow old; they may die of old age, but they die young.

W. Pinero

The grand essentials to happiness in this life are something to do, something to love and something to hope for.

Joseph Addison

*"Hold fast to dreams,
For if dreams die
Life is a broken-winged bird,
That cannot fly."*

Langston Hughes

And I really like this one:

Growing old is mandatory; growing up is optional...

Thanks

I need to thank many people for the love and kindnesses they have shown me during the last nine weeks. First and foremost among these is Ingrid, my dear wife of forty-five years. She was with me every step of the way. She accompanied me to all of the initial doctor visits and came with me on those days when procedures were performed, because we feared that some of them might make it impossible for me to drive home by myself. She spoiled me throughout the treatment period, like serving me breakfast in bed, when I had another one of those sleepless nights, when I spent as much time in the bathroom as in the bedroom.

I also want to thank my children and their families and all of my other relatives and friends for the many prayers and good wishes they have sent my way.

A special "thank you" goes out to all of the medical people who were involved in treating the disease that has invaded my body – Dr. Bauer, who immediately recognized that something irregular was taking place within me and who initiated the next important step; Dr. Delgado, who performed the biopsy and discussed the implications of these findings with me; Dr. Sinclair, who did all of the preparatory work needed for the actual radiation therapy to take place. I could not have wished for a better team of doctors to be involved in my case.

I thank Petra, the dietitian, for the sound advice she gave me concerning my diet during the treatment period and for the rest of my life.

Although I did not have all that much personal contact with Roseanne, the office manager, I thank her for her willingness to look over the manuscript of this story.

I thank Jan, the nurse, and Tina, the medical assistant, for efficiently and cheerfully dealing with me: weigh-ins, blood pressure readings, prescriptions, urine tests, etc.

A special "thank you" goes to Megan, the receptionist. She was the first person I saw when I came in and the last person I saw when I went out. Her warm smile and friendly greetings and goodbyes started and ended each visit in the most pleasant manner.

I most sincerely thank Pat, the chief therapist. She explained that which lay before me in a most professional and sensitive manner. She also performed, assisted by Brenda, the critical work done in the CT room – the scanning, marker placement and the dye injection into the bladder. When some time later I asked her how the dye was actually brought into the bladder (I imagined an elevated drip bag and a lengthy tube inserted through the urethra all the way into the bladder), she showed me the syringe, about five inches long and two inches thick, with an adapter tip, with which two ounces of the liquid are actually propelled into the bladder. This is done twice for a total of four ounces of the water/dye solution. I asked Pat if she would look over my manuscript to see whether I got the technical details of the various procedures right. She agreed, and I thank her for that, too.

My most personal relationship, however, was developed with the three therapists whom I saw every day during the treatment period – Ted, Brenda and Donna. I call them the "Keepers of the Vault." Each morning there was a friendly greeting and I always felt as if they were happy to see me. They performed their work in a most

112

professional and efficient manner, and by the way they made everything look so easy and natural, they demonstrated (at least to me) how really good they are at what they do. I was also glad that they willingly and enthusiastically answered all of the questions I had for them. Upon my request, they showed me how the table is slid toward the linear accelerator, how it is then raised to be on the level of the openings on the side walls and the foot end wall. They let me see how the light beams coming from these three openings are aligned so that the rays of light emanating from them form a cross over the "tattoo" on each of the upper thighs and the groin area. They told me that the radiation comes from a garbage can sized container inside the massive accelerator, how it is swirled around, and then sent onto the patient's body. It was also explained to me that the rotating part of the machine moves 179 degrees down on one side and then down on the other side – it does not go all the way around. I also learned that the machine is never really shut down, but that it does take twelve minutes every morning to get it into its working mode. I liked the fact that they were so willing and eager to explain all this to me. I cannot help but think that perhaps the three of them were appreciative of the fact that someone had come along who was interested in how everything worked and in the important work that they are doing. I thank them for sharing their experiences and their knowledge with me. But more than that, I thank them for being the wonderful people that they are.

And Now ....

And now I will joyfully go on with my life, eager to experience all that still lies before me, for I know that...

There are still so many wonderful places to see

So many good books to read

So much beautiful music to hear

So many new friends to meet.

God Bless

Peace and Love

Helmut

About the Author, Helmut Stefan

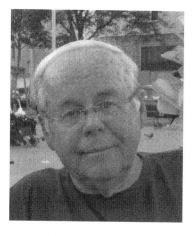

Helmut Stefan is a retired Chicago public school teacher who loves to travel, read and write.

In 1998 he was awarded a National Endowment for the Humanities Fellowship to study "Mozart, the Man, his Music and his Vienna." Classical music, especially the music of W. A. Mozart, is one of the great passions of his life.

He and his wife Ingrid and their grown children live in the Chicago area.

Other books by Helmut Stefan:

Trio in D minor

Feathers in the Wind

Made in the USA
Charleston, SC
12 April 2015